W9-BGA-531

The

Blueprints

of

Infection

Student Manual

DEVELOPED BY
EDUCATION DEVELOPMENT CENTER, INC.

KENDALL/HUNT PUBLISHING COMPANY
4050 Westmark Drive P.O. Box 1840 Dubuque, Iowa 52004-1840

This book was prepared with the support of National Science Foundation (NSF) Grant
ESI-9255722. However, any opinions, findings, conclusions and/or recommendations
herein are those of the author and do not necessarily reflect the view of NSF.

Library of Congress Catalog Card Number: 96-80038

ISBN 0-7872-2207-0

Printed in the United States of America
10 9 8 7 6 5 4 3 2 1

EDC   Education
Development
Center, Inc.

CENTER FOR SCIENCE EDUCATION

Dear Students:

Welcome to *Insights in Biology*. In this module, *The Blueprints of Infection,* you will be exploring the causes and modes of transmission of infectious diseases. Your study of infectious agents, such as viruses and bacteria, will also provide insight into basic biological processes including how these agents disrupt normal cellular functions and how the immune system responds to infectious agents. Organisms may be infectious because of information encoded in their DNA or they may disrupt the transfer and expression of the proteins which are encoded in DNA. One of the storylines of this module is the infectious disease, cholera. You will begin your study as a disease detective, gather information on cholera and other diseases and finish as a role player in a Colombian town trying to develop an action plan to stem their cholera epidemic. All the complexities of decision-making in the modern world will be explored in this role play.

Glance through the pages of this manual. Your first instinct is correct: This is not a traditional biology textbook. Although textbooks provide a good deal of useful information, they are not the only way to discover science. In this Student Manual, you will find that chapters have been replaced by Learning Experiences that include readings and activities. The activities include laboratory experimentation, role playing, concept mapping, model building, simulation exercises, and a research project. These learning experiences emphasize the processes of science and the connections among biological concepts.

One of our main goals is to engage you in the excitement of biology. The study of biology is much more than facts. It is a discipline that is as alive as the subjects it portrays: new questions arise, new theories are proposed, and new understandings are achieved. As a result of these new insights, technologies are developed which will impact your everyday lives and the kinds of decisions you will need to make. We hope that this curriculum encourages you to ask questions, to develop greater problem-solving and thinking skills, and to recognize the importance of science in your life.

Insights in Biology Staff

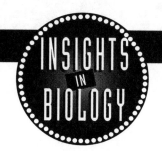

TABLE OF **C**ONTENTS

LEARNING **E**XPERIENCES

APPENDIX

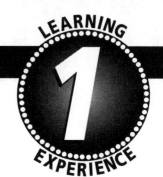

DISEASE DETECTIVES

PROLOGUE

. . . During an epidemic of 1918, according to medical lore, victims were struck down almost in midstride. Four women in a bridge group played cards together until 11 o'clock in the evening. By the next morning, three of them were dead. One man got on a streetcar feeling well enough to go to work, rode six blocks and died. During the single month of October, [this epidemic killed] 196,000 people in this country—more than twice as many as would die of AIDS during the first 10 years of that epidemic...

Excerpted from Robin Marantz Henig, "Flu Pandemic." The New York Times Magazine, *November 29, 1992.*

Who were the victims? What set them apart from those who remained healthy? What caused all these deaths? Scientists, researchers, doctors, and public health officials study outbreaks of disease in order to understand how each disease is spread, what is causing it, and how to stop it. In the case of the people described above, did anyone know how the disease spread? Could anything have been done to prevent it? How did the disease actually kill? We know now that by the end of the winter of 1918–1919, two billion persons around the world had come down with influenza, also known as the flu, and between 20 and 40 million had suddenly died from a disease that seems common today. If it happened once, could it happen again?

In this first learning experience, you will examine one of the early stories in the development of our understanding of infectious disease. Major discoveries in this field, providing fundamental insight into how living organisms function, began with John Snow, an English surgeon. These discoveries have also led to greater understanding in the control of disease and the maintenance of good health. John Snow traced cases of an outbreak of the highly infectious disease cholera in an effort to find the source. Using the following reading and excerpts from John Snow's writings, you will retrace this man's steps as he discovered preliminary answers to many of the questions about the source of the outbreak, who was affected, and what could be done to break the chain of transmission of disease.

Figure 1.1
Flu epidemic

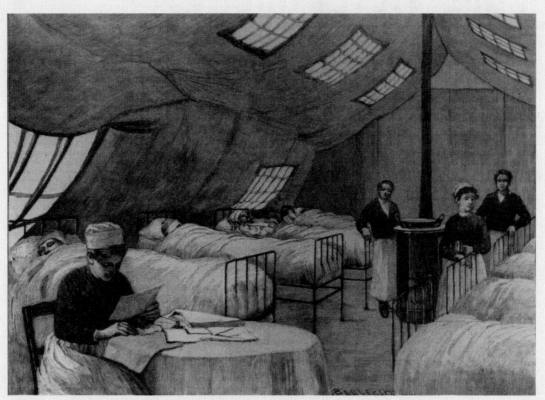

L'ÉPIDÉMIE D'INFLUENZA. —Vue intérieure de la tente-hôpital.

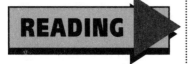

CHOLERA

In the early 1800s, England was in the throes of the industrial revolution. Until the late 1700s, most of England's workers lived in the countryside, laboring as farmers. But by 1830, the economic heart of England was in its cities where laborers, forced off of their farms, were competing for low wages in the new factory economy. Market towns could not change quickly enough to keep pace with their expanding populations. Cities had not yet invented police forces, and fire brigades services had to be bought. Housing was overcrowded. Because there was no system for collecting garbage, it piled up in streets, creating a breeding ground for vermin. Usually, raw sewage was thrown into the streets or into the nearest stream, which might be a source of drinking water. No city had an adequate clean water supply as yet. Of course, there was no gas or electric lighting at that time. In short, the infrastructure of the modern city had yet to be invented.

By 1830, the upper and lower social classes were divided dramatically. While the desperately poor laborers struggled each day just to feed and clothe themselves, the newly rich factory owners who employed them were managing the world's most powerful empire for England and for their own profit. Poor laborers, who were paid starvation wages, feared and mistrusted the wealthy classes. In 1798, observing the overcrowding and miserable conditions in England's new cities, the economist Thomas Malthus had written about the population explosion and argued that the growth in population guaranteed that poverty and starvation would become a severe problem.

The growing number of city-dwellers created a sudden increase in the demand for medical workers. At the same time, Britain's medical students were first being required to learn about human anatomy. To help institute this requirement, the dissection of a cadaver (a human corpse) was included in the required curriculum of medical schools. The only legal source of cadavers at that time was executed criminals, and unfortunately for medical students, the number of students far outnumbered the men and women who had been hanged from the gallows. So, medical schools began hiring grave robbers to provide them with an additional supply of corpses. Most of the graves poached were graves of the indigent. To the poor, it looked as though doctors used the bodies of the underclass to do their training, then used their training to benefit the upper class.

In 1832, Parliament passed the Anatomy Act, which provided doctors with the unclaimed bodies of people who had died in workhouses, prisons, and hospitals. This law guaranteed that all the cadavers for dissection would be poor. Poor people could not afford the services of doctors. For most of the working class, the only contact they could expect to have with a doctor happened if they were stricken in an epidemic and forcibly dragged to an unsanitary public hospital for "treatment;" in that case, they could expect to die in the hospital. With the passage of the Anatomy Act, it appeared to many of Britain's poor that the rich medical doctors were going to add insult to injury by interfering with their traditional, religious burial—literally by robbing their graves for "science." While the poor mistrusted the motives of the medical profession and the rest of the "better" classes, the educated upper classes generally saw the attitudes of the poor towards the medical profession as proof of their ignorance and irrationality.

In 1826, a *pandemic* (a disease occurring among many individuals worldwide, in contrast to an *epidemic,* a disease that occurs among individuals locally) of the dreaded disease cholera had begun in India. It was observed there by British physicians and tracked as it made its way first to Russia by 1830, then to the Austro-Hungarian Empire by 1831.

Cholera killed 100,000 people along the Danube River before making its way into Western Europe. Then, in 1832, in the same year that the Anatomy Act was passed, the cholera disease found its way to the shores of Britain.

At first, the reports of cholera aggravated English class tensions. Doctors reported that in Europe, cholera's victims were generally from the poorer classes. Conspiracy theories emerged. Some believed that cholera was a big profiteering hoax, drummed up by the grave-robbing doctors to scare people into buying medicine. Others believed that cholera was not a disease at all. They thought the government (which was, after all, in the hands of England's wealthiest citizens) had decided to poison the wells of the poor, to kill the "surplus population" which Malthus had predicted.

Gruesome descriptions of the disease helped to fuel the panic and mistrust. Many victims died rapidly after experiencing terrifying symptoms. Often, the victim would feel absolutely healthy one minute, and the next, feel extremely nauseated. This nausea would be followed by a sudden and total evacuation of the bowels. From here, the victim would have the sensation of a great weight around the waist and a prickly sensation in arms and legs. Cold, clammy sweats would begin, together with a suppressed pulse and severe headache. Within one

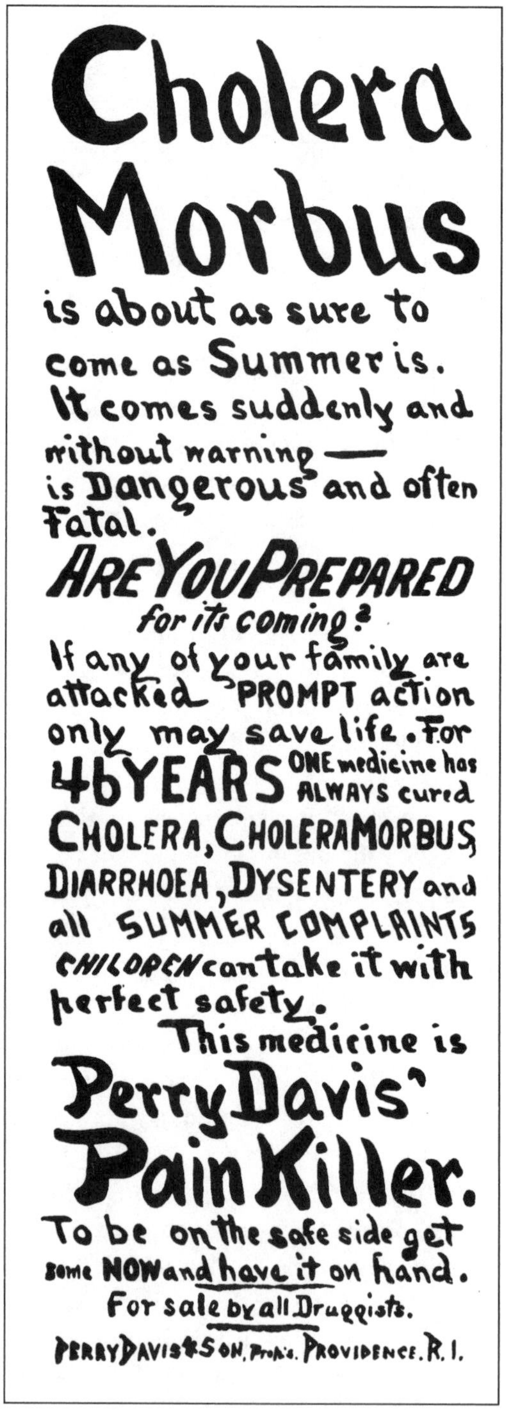

Figure 1.2
Was there a cure? "Morbus" was a synonym for "disease."

hour of the disease's onset, a person's bowel movements would produce an odorless liquid, filled with rice-like pellets (doctors later determined that this "rice" was actually fragments of the victim's intestinal lining). Soon, the patient's body would shrink and shrivel. Acute cramps would begin in the fingers and toes and then spread to the rest of the body. Skin would turn blue or black. Death generally occurred within two to seven days.

No one knew the cause of the disease, but doctors had a variety of theories. Some believed that it was carried on the air by an unhealthy "effluvia." These "effluvyists" suggested that the effluvia was exhaled by those who were already ill. Others, "miasmatists," believed that the garbage and feces covering streets of the overcrowded cities produced some kind of deadly vapor or miasma which, when inhaled, caused the cholera. Other theorists believed that an unhealthy diet was the cause. Still other beliefs included unclean water, or the "immoral drunkenness" and "dirty habits" of the poor. Some suggested that there might be a chemical contaminant causing the illness. Some said the disease was a punishment from God, and that there was nothing to be done to stop it.

It was in this social and scientific context that John Snow, in 1832, an 18-year-old surgeon's apprentice, had his first experiences comforting the dying victims of cholera.

After the 1832 pandemic, cholera did not return to Britain until 1848. By the time it returned, Snow had become one of the most famous surgeons in England. He had become a leading pioneer in the use of surgical anesthetics (a brand new invention), and had become a personal physician of Queen Victoria. In the sixteen years since 1832, the class tensions in England had, if anything, become worse. The medical profession was still arguing over the causes of cholera and the public's feelings about it had not improved. But one major new idea had been introduced to the medical world. Though no one had yet proved it, a few radicals were suggesting that some diseases might be caused by microbes. John Snow knew of this idea, and he thought it might be true.

▶ ANALYSIS

1. Consider the conditions which existed in England in the 1830s. What do you think contributed to the outbreak of cholera?

2. Give some reasons why most cholera victims came from the lower class.

3. Why do you think the cholera epidemic stopped in 1832?

4. The cholera pandemic began in India in 1826. How do you think a disease spreads across continents and around the world? Do you think this happens today? More or less frequently? Why?

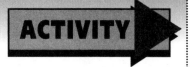

ACTIVITY

Investigating the Nature and Cause of Cholera

INTRODUCTION   John Snow had three opportunities to study cholera: first in the pandemic of 1832, again in the epidemic of 1848–1849, and finally in the epidemic of 1853–1854. In 1854 he published "On the Mode of the Communication of Cholera," in which he outlined all of his discoveries. In his work, Snow presented the evidence he had collected and then used that evidence to draw conclusions.

You are going to begin a scientific analysis of data in order to solve the mystery of cholera by examining precisely the same evidence that was available to Snow in 1854. You will be reading six separate sets of excerpts from Snow's writing. As you read the data sets, think about the following:

- To solve the mystery as Snow did, you will have to use the tools of 1854. You will have no microscope.

- In one respect, your job will be far easier than Snow's. Snow had to collect all of the evidence, sort through it, and figure out which evidence was relevant to his study. All you have to do is examine the evidence that he had already determined to be relevant, and analyze it.

- When Snow began, he had already heard two decades of medical debate about the possible causes of cholera. Like many scientists, he began with a hypothesis. Then he went out to find the evidence necessary to test his hypothesis.

In John Snow's day, doctors were searching for the answers to several crucial questions:

1. How did cholera spread?
    - Were the effluvia or miasma theories correct?
    - Was the disease spread by some other means?
    - Could the disease spread by a variety of methods?

2. Why did some of the people exposed to victims of cholera get sick, while others did not? Why were the poor especially vulnerable to the disease?

3. Could the spread of cholera be prevented? If so, how?

4. Once a person had cholera, could he or she be treated? If so, how? (John Snow did *not* discover the answer to this question. It was answered later by other researchers. But by the end of this learning experience, you should be able to make an educated guess (*hypothesis*) about the answer to this question.)

5. What was the *underlying* cause of the disease? (John Snow could not prove his answer to this question, but he made an educated guess that turned out to be correct. What do you suppose he hypothesized?)

▶ TASK

Read Data Set 1. After reading it, stop and fill in the Data Analysis chart by completing the following two steps.

1. Determine which of the questions listed can be answered using the information given in the Data Set you have just read. Then, write the answers that can be derived from the data in the row labeled "hypothesis." In other words, answer the questions with your own hypotheses (possibly your hypotheses will be similar to those developed by Snow). If a question is not addressed in the data set put N/A for "not applicable" in the appropriate box below the question.

2. Think carefully about the information from the excerpted data. If possible, show how the data presented so far are inconclusive. In other words, even if the data point toward a particular answer to any of the five questions, other answers might still be possible. Look for these "holes" in the proof of your hypothesis and record your ideas in the row labeled "Reasons data may be inconclusive."

Proceed to the second data set, read it, and fill in that part of the chart. You may need to refer back to material you have already read. Follow the same procedure until you have finished Data Set 6.

SNOW ON CHOLERA

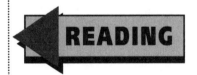

Excerpts adapted from the original, as reprinted in How We Know: An Explanation of the Scientific Process, *by Martin Goldstein and Inge F. Goldstein, Plenum Press, NY, 1978.*

DATA SET 1 When it appears on a fresh island or continent, cholera always strikes first at a seaport.

It travels along highly populated areas, never going faster than people travel, and generally much more slowly.

It never attacks the crew of a ship sailing away from a country that is free of cholera.

DATA SET 2 I called recently to ask about the death of Mrs. Gore, the wife of a labourer, from cholera, at New Leigham Road, Streatham. I found that a son of the deceased had been living and working at Chelsea. He came home ill with a bowel complaint, of which he died in a day or two. His death took place on August 18th. His mother, who attended to him, was taken ill on the next day, and died the day following (August 20th). There were no other deaths from cholera registered in any of the metropolitan districts, until the 26th of August, within two or three miles of the above place . . .

* * *

John Barnes, aged 39, an agricultural labourer, became severely ill on the 28th of December 1832; he had been suffering from diarrhea and cramps for two days previously. He was visited by Mr. George Hopps, a respectable surgeon at Redhouse, who finding him sinking into collapse, requested an interview with his brother, Mr. J. Hopps of York. This experienced practitioner at once recognized the case as one of Asiatic cholera . . . He immediately began investigating for some probable source of contagion, but in vain; no such source could be discovered.

While the surgeons were vainly trying to discover where the disease could possibly have come from, the mystery was all at once, and most unexpectedly, unraveled by the arrival in the village of the son of the shoemaker, living at Leeds. He informed the surgeons that his uncle's wife (his father's sister) had died of cholera two weeks before that time, and that as she had no children, her clothes had been sent to Monkton by a common carrier. The clothes had not been washed; Barnes had opened the box in the evening; on the next day he had fallen sick of the disease.

During the illness of Mrs. Barnes, [the wife of John Barnes: she and two friends who visited Barnes during his illness also got cholera], her mother, who was living at Tockwith, a healthy village 5 miles distant from Monkton, was asked to attend her. She went to Monkton accordingly, remained with her daughter for 2 days, washed her daughter's linen, and set out on her return home, apparently in good health. While in the act of walking home she was seized with the malady and fell down in collapse on the road. She was carried home to her cottage and placed by the side of her bedridden husband. He, and also the daughter who lived with them, got ill. All three died within 2 days. Only one other case occurred in the village of Tockwith, and it was not a fatal case . . .

It would be easy by going through the medical journals and works that have been published on cholera, to quote enough cases similar to the above to fill a large volume.

* * *

Nothing has been found to favor the spread of cholera more than a lack of personal cleanliness, whether arising from habit or a shortage of water . . . The bed linen nearly always becomes wetted by the cholera evacuations, and as these do not have the usual color and odor of diarrhea, the hands of the person waiting on the patient [usually a woman, in England in 1850] become soiled without their knowing it. Unless these persons are scrupulously clean in their habits, and wash their hands before taking food, they must accidentally swallow some of the excretion and leave some on the food they handle or prepare, which has to be eaten by the rest of the family who, amongst the working classes, often have to take their meals in the sick room. Hence the thousands of instances in which, amongst their class of the population, a case of cholera in one member of the family is followed by other cases, whilst medical men and others, who merely visit the patients, generally escape . . .

On the other hand, the duties performed about the body, such as laying it out (for the funeral), when done by women of the working class, who make the occasion one of eating and drinking, are often followed by an attack of cholera . . .

*** * ***

When, on the other hand, cholera is introduced into the better kind of houses . . . it hardly ever spreads from one member of the family to another. The wealthy constantly use the hand-basin and towel, and their kitchens and bedrooms are separated.

DATA SET 3   Cholera invariably begins with the affliction of the (digestive) canal. The disease often proceeds with so little feeling of general illness, that the patient does not consider himself in danger, or even [ask] for advice, till the [illness] is far advanced . . .

In all the cases of cholera that I have attended, the loss of fluid from the stomach and bowels has been sufficient to account for death, when the poor diet and health of the patient was taken into account, together with the suddenness of the diarrhea, and the fact that the process of absorption of water in the digestive tract appears to be suspended during the illness.

A period of time passes between the time when the cholera poison enters the system, and the beginning of the illness. This period is called the period of incubation.

DATA SET 4   In 1849, there were in Thomas Street, Horseleydown, two rows of houses close together consisting of a number of small houses or cottages inhabited by poor people. The houses of the two rows were back to back . . . with a separating space between them, divided into small back yards in which were located the outhouses of both the courts. These outhouses drained into the same trench that flowed out to an open sewer that passed by the far end of both house rows. In one row of buildings, the cholera committed fearful devastation, while in the adjoining row, there was only one fatality and one milder case of the disease. In the former row of houses, the slops of dirty water poured down by the inhabitants into a channel in front of the houses and got into the well from which they obtained their water. In the latter houserow, water was obtained from a different well.

* * *

Dr. Thomas King Chambers informed me that at Ilford in Essex in the summer of 1849, the cholera prevailed very severely in a row of houses a little way from the main part of the town. It had visited every house in the row but one. The refuse which overflowed from the out-houses and a pigsty could be seen running into the well over the surface of the ground, and the water had a nasty smell, yet it was used by all the people in the houses except for the one woman who escaped the cholera. That house was inhabited by a woman who took in linen to wash, and she, finding that the water gave the linen an offensive smell, paid a person to fetch water for her from the pump in the town, and this water she used for culinary purposes as well as for washing.

READING ▶

THE INVESTIGATION CONTINUES

What are your ideas about the evidence presented so far? Do you feel it is adequate to answer accurately the questions posed at the beginning of the Task? John Snow did not feel he had enough evidence. He therefore carried out the following two separate experiments, which revolutionized medicine. Think about the following as you read the next two Data Sets.

– What does the information Snow collected prove?

– What holes remain in the data which are needed to support the hypothesis?

DATA SET 5   In 1849, a particularly terrible outbreak of cholera occurred along Broad Street, near Golden Square, in London. Over a 10-day period, almost 500 people died there within 250 yards of the intersections of Broad and Cambridge streets. At this intersection, there was a particularly popular public water pump—well known for the good taste of its water. By the time of this catastrophe, based upon the anecdotal evidence summarized in Data Sets 1–4, Snow was more or less certain that cholera could be transmitted through the water supply. He believed that the water at the Broad Street pump must have been contaminated.

To prove his hunch, he went to the London General Register Office and got the names and addresses of the 83 people whose deaths had been recorded there. Then, going door to door, he collected information about the water-drinking habits of all the cholera victims in the area. He produced the following chart:

83 deaths					
73 living near Broad Street pump			10 not living near pump		
61	6	6	5	3	2
Known to have drunk pump water	Believed not to have drunk pump water	No information	In families sending to pump for water	Children attending school near pump	No information

Snow next gave two sets of data that strongly support the role of the pump. There were two groups of people living near the Broad Street pump who had very few cases of cholera: the inhabitants of a workhouse (where homeless people were housed and given labor to do—as Oliver Twist was) and the employees of a brewery. Snow interviewed the manager of the brewery and discovered that the brewery gave free beer to its employees and had its own well. The manager was certain that his employees did not, in fact, use the Broad Street pump at all.

As soon as Snow informed the city officials of his data, they had the handle of the Broad Street pump removed. By this time, the cholera epidemic had more or less died down of its own accord. But the simple act of removing the pump handle was the first time in world history that a public health measure was taken as a direct response to scientific data.

DATA SET 6

Finally, in the epidemic of 1853–1854, Snow performed one more experiment. In London at this time, there was still no public water supply. However, since 1832, the city had grown tremendously, and entrepreneurs had begun to sell water door to door. Water companies ran pipes (sometimes wooden; sometimes lead) along streets in some neighborhoods, and the residents could buy water that was brought through these pipes. If a homeowner bought the water, a pipe would be run from the street main

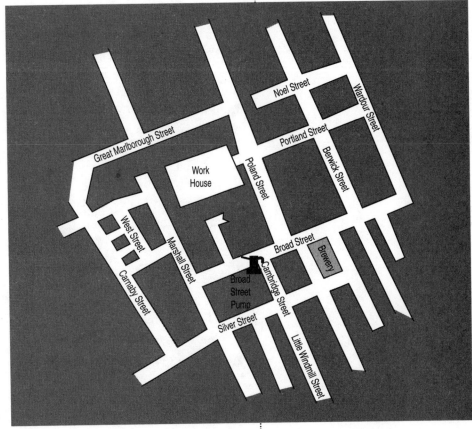

Figure 1.3
Map of the Broad Street area

into the front entrance of the home. This was much more convenient than having to run to the neighborhood pump as people had done on Broad Street. In many neighborhoods, two different companies competed door to door to sell their water. Thus, Snow could compare the relationship between water supply and cholera deaths both in different neighborhoods and within similar neighborhoods.

Snow did a tremendous amount of work, going door to door to see if there was a relationship between the type of water a person drank and their risk of getting cholera. The results of his work were summarized in the following chart:

	Number of houses	Death from cholera	Deaths per 10,000 houses
Southwark & Vauxhall Co.	40,046	1,263	315
Lambeth Company	26,107	98	37
Rest of London	256,423	1,422	59

Based upon the chart, Snow went on to calculate the death rate per 10,000 for those persons receiving their water from the Southwark and Vauxhall Co. and the death rate for those persons receiving their water from the Lambeth Co. See if you can make the calculations yourself. What do you conclude?

It turned out that after the 1849 epidemic, the Lambeth Company had moved the intake for its water pipes to a part of the Thames River upstream from where London's sewage poured into the river. The Southwark and Vauxhall Co. had not—its pipes still brought in water containing London sewage.

▶ ANALYSIS

1. In the clearest language possible, write a hypothesis about how cholera spread. Using all the information accumulated by John Snow up to 1854, explain how these data support your hypothesis.

2. After 1854, what important questions still remained to be answered about cholera?

3. Describe how you might go about conducting a study to determine the cause of the disease in the following fictional community. Include what you would need to see, the questions you would ask, and data you might collect.

Desiduous is a small town, famous for its Desiduous Pickles. However, in 1991, economic times were tough. Recession meant less money and less money meant fewer pickles on the American plate. Economic problems were nothing new to Desiduous, whose town motto was, "As goes the American economy, so goes the pickle."

On Monday, July 20, however, Desiduous' distress was more than economic. Two previously healthy prominent male citizens, ages 35 and 42, had died mysteriously within twenty-four hours and panic flowed through the town like juice from a shattered pickle jar.

Roscoe Clayman, the owner of the town multiplex theater, was a respected bowler and avid tuba player. Reginald Willowslip was unemployed, a retired pickle taster in the local factory who kept his taste buds in shape at the local saloons and pubs. The only thing these two men seemed to have in common was being avid philatelists. Both had recently attended the Annual Stamp Collectors' Convention in Topeka, held at the beautiful and elegant Colossus Hotel.

In fact, across Kansas at this time, stamp collectors were falling ill and dying at an alarming rate. Within a three week period, 183 cases of the so-called Stamp Collectors' Syndrome were reported. After the first week of this apparent outbreak/epidemic, the Centers for Disease Control agency in Atlanta was contacted and six young and eager epidemiologists rushed to the scene to begin intensive and extensive investigations.

EPILOGUE

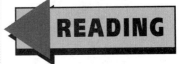
READING

It is appropriate that a discussion of the nature of disease begins with the story of John Snow. In fact, this is true for two reasons: First, Snow's work was a pioneering effort to combine scientific medical inquiry with statistics—already a critical innovation in the history of science and medicine. Second, Snow's study is one of the first recorded in the field of *epidemiology*, a discipline that documents epidemics and attempts to determine the causes. Snow's research is also a proper place to begin our study of disease.

During the time of John Snow, cities lacked public sewage systems and clean water supplies. They also lacked police departments, fire departments, paved road systems, gas, and electricity; in other words, the urban world of the early industrial revolution was a dirty, chaotic place. Unless one had the money to purchase these services through a private company, life in the city was a dismal prospect.

But Snow's work was a catalyst to change all of this. Once there was scientific, statistical proof linking disease to dirty drinking water and untreated sewage, tremendous new pressures were placed upon city governments to manage these problems. To build city-wide sewage disposal and treatment systems meant that the city governments in Europe and the United States had to be better organized. Taxes had to be raised to pay for new construction projects. A chain reaction began. Once city governments began to take responsibility for sewage and water, it was a natural step to garbage collection, police and fire protection, and other services the industrialized world now takes so much for granted that we refer to them as "basic services."

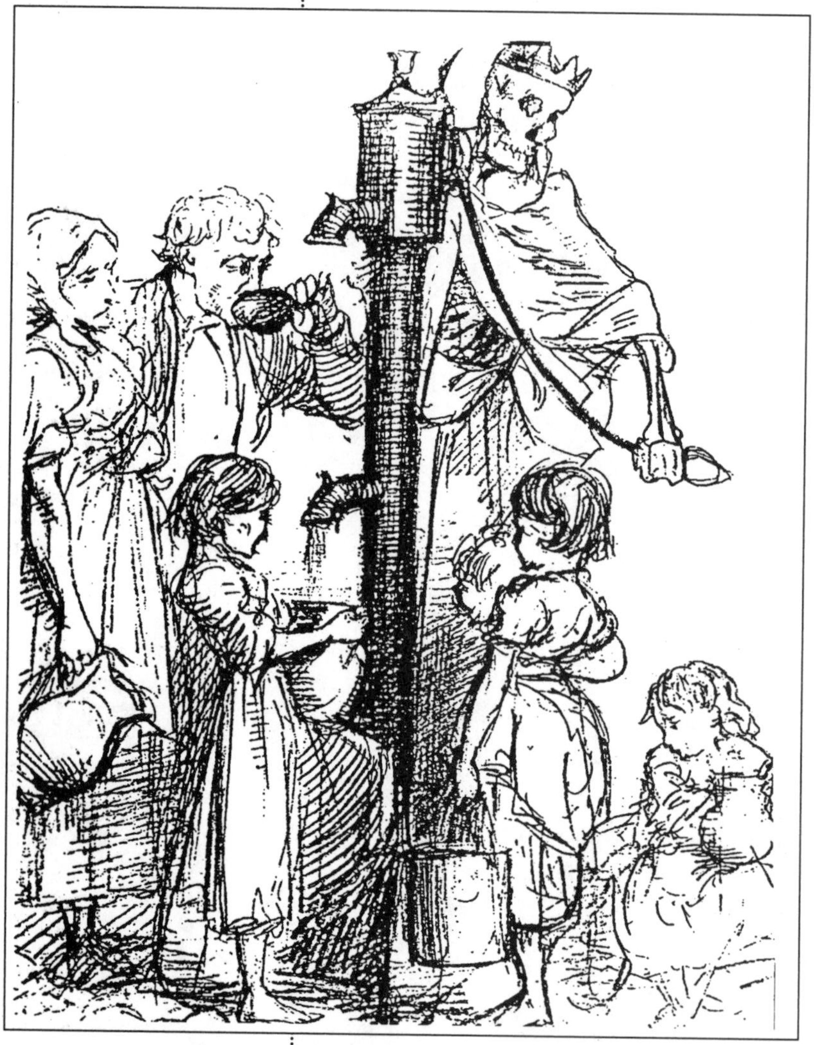

The introduction of these infrastructure systems, making urban life better for everyone, reduced some of the class tensions in Britain. Finally, medicine and government made some changes that tangibly improved the lives of the working classes. Tensions did not disappear, but by the late 19th century, the unhealthy and miserable conditions of the urban poor had been substantially reduced.

Today, it is hard for Americans to imagine life without these "necessities." Just 140 years ago, it was hard for most people to imagine life with them. Infrastructure has changed the deepest fabric of our lives. But to suppose that such changes have been universal would be naive. While the vast majority of Americans no longer have to worry about the risk of cholera, outbreaks of the scourge continue to occur around the world. In much of the world, the wealth needed to build even the most rudimentary water supply and sewage disposal systems is lacking. Indeed, recent outbreaks of cholera in Latin America and Africa have spurred massive new efforts to build such infrastructure in many of the countries where these outbreaks occurred. Perhaps history is repeating itself.

Figure 1.4
"Death's Dispensary" by George John Pinwell, 1866, reproduced with permission from Philadelphia Museum of Art: SmithKline Beecham Corporation Fund.

EXTENDING IDEAS

▶ Read stories about other disease detectives. Compare one of these stories to John Snow's story including the society in which it occurred, the evidence, the techniques used, prior knowledge of the researcher, and what the impact of the discovery was on the spread of disease. The powerful story of HIV, for example, is described in numerous books, magazines and newspaper articles.

▶ Find out what the Centers for Disease Control and Prevention (CDC) agency does, what its role is, what techniques they use, and what kinds of jobs people do in the organization.

ON THE JOB

WATER POLLUTION CONTROL TECHNICIANS   Are you concerned with the quality of the water you drink or the air you breathe? Pollution control technicians conduct tests and field investigations to determine ways to both monitor and control the contamination of freshwater, of the air, or the soil. Two major specialties of technicians are water pollution control and air pollution control. Although some technicians may specialize in noise, light or soil pollution. Water pollution control technicians help identify sources of water pollution and ways to reduce it. They collect water samples and perform physical and chemical tests in order to collect data such as temperature and turbidity; streak plates to determine the concentration of bacterial contaminants; record results; and read and interpret charts, graphs and tables. Technicians usually have an understanding of the usual environment (the air, water, soil, and so on) in which the data is collected in order to detect the presence of gases or particles which are not normally present and discriminate between the importance of pollution factors. Technicians usually have either a two year college degree in physical sciences or two year post high school training in pollution control technology. Since this is a relatively new field, some positions with on-the-job training are available to those with a high school diploma and appropriate experience. Classes such as mathematics, chemistry, physics, biology (conservation or ecology), computer courses, and English are recommended.

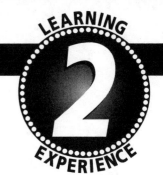
Epidemic!

PROLOGUE **E**ven before John Snow made his methodical, scientific study of how cholera spread, people were aware that certain illnesses could be passed from one individual to another. Avoiding contact with sick people, fumigating homes where sickness had occurred, and burning bedding and clothing of sick individuals were common practices. In this learning experience, you will be examining the many ways that diseases can be transmitted; you will then determine what, if anything, can be done to break the chain of transmission.

The End of the World is Nigh

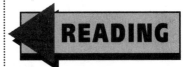

READING

The various outbreaks of cholera in London and other cities such as New York and Boston during the 1800s are examples of a phenomenon known as an epidemic. An outbreak of a disease is considered an epidemic when it is prevalent and spreads rapidly among many individuals in a community at the same time. Epidemics of a disease that occur simultaneously around the world are considered pandemics. Epidemics and pandemics are part of life and of history. Some examples of these, past and present, are shown in Table 2.2 on the following page.

Since Snow's time, epidemiologists (individuals who study the pattern and occurrence of outbreaks of disease) and other scientists have determined that disease can be carried from one individual to another by a variety of methods, called *modes of transmission*. These include spread resulting from direct, person-to-person contact or touching; from contaminated water and food (as Snow determined); through the air; and through the saliva or feces of insects or other animals (called *vectors*). With the knowledge of how a disease is transmitted (communicated), perhaps measures can be taken to reduce its spread or to avoid it ourselves.

Figure 2.1
Diseases such as a cold may be spread when saliva droplets are sprayed into the air during a sneeze.

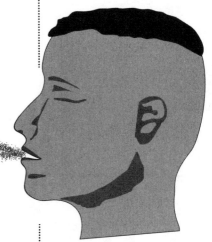

In general, specific diseases are spread by only one mode of transmission; for example, flu is spread when saliva from an infected person is sprayed into the air during a sneeze and is considered an airborne disease. Table 2.2 indicates how certain diseases are spread.

Table 2.2
Epidemics and pandemics through history

DISEASE	MODE OF TRANSMISSION	LOCATION/DATE (A.D.)	INFECTION RATE AND/OR DEATH TOLL
smallpox	direct contact	Roman Empire (165–180)	25%–35% of population affected
bubonic plague	fleas on rats (vector)	Europe (1347–1350)	17–28 million deaths; 33%–50% of population affected
influenza	airborne	worldwide (1918–1919)	2 million deaths
polio	contaminated water	U.S. (1943–1956)	22,000 deaths; 400,000 affected
tuberculosis	airborne	worldwide (ongoing)	500,000 deaths annually
diarrheal diseases (primarily enteric (intestinal) bacteria and rotavirus)	contaminated food and water	developing countries (South America, Africa, Asia) (ongoing)	10 million deaths annually
malaria	mosquitoes	developing countries (South America, Africa, Asia) (ongoing)	1.2 million deaths annually
AIDS	direct contact	worldwide (ongoing)	25–30 million reported infections

▶ **ANALYSIS**

In preparation for a discussion, write responses to these questions in your notebook.

1. How do modes of transmission of the infectious diseases listed in Table 2.2 differ?

2. Through what kinds of activities might individuals come in contact with each of these diseases?

3. What are ways people might try to avoid contracting these diseases?

4. List any infectious and noninfectious diseases that have occurred in your community during the past year. For each one, describe how you think it was communicated (transmitted).

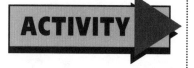

OUTBREAK

INTRODUCTION   In this investigation, you will participate in an epidemic without suffering any dire consequences. You will spread an "infection" by using one mode of transmission—direct contact. Then, using a standard technique in the field of microbiology (the study of microorganisms), you will be able to "diagnose" the presence of the infection and discover who has been "infected." As you analyze your data, think about the kinds of preventative measures that might be used to halt the spread of this infection.

▶ MATERIALS NEEDED

For each student:
- 1 pair of safety goggles
- 1 sterile cotton swab or inoculating loop
- 1 nutrient agar plate

For each group of eight students:
- 1 piece of contaminated candy (hard candy)
- 1 wax marking pencil (grease pencil)
- 1 test tube containing nutrient broth

For the class:
- soap, detergent, or disinfectant
- warm water
- 4 sponges
- yeast solution
- sterilized tweezers or tongs

▶ PROCEDURE

1. Count off within your group and write your number on an agar plate.

2. Wash your hands thoroughly. ***NOTE:*** When working with microorganisms, certain practices should be followed in order to ensure that the materials you are working with do not become contaminated with microorganisms present in the air, on your hands and clothing, and on working surfaces. These practices are known as *sterile* or *aseptic* techniques. Sterile techniques also protect the investigator from becoming contaminated by the materials he/she is working with. Although all of the organisms you will be working with are harmless, sterile techniques should still be used. These include:
   - Wash hands thoroughly with soap and water before starting and at the conclusion of the experiment;
   - Wash the laboratory table with disinfectant or detergent before and after the experiment;
   - Use sterile media, glassware, and tools;
   - Keep hands away from working ends of tools (such as inoculating loops, cotton swabs, and tweezers) and glassware. Do not touch the insides of agar plates;
   - Keep bottles, tubes, and flasks covered when not in use;
   - Do not mouth pipette;
   - Do not eat, drink, or smoke in the work area.

SAFETY NOTE: *Always wear safety goggles when conducting experiments.*

3. If your number is 1, the instructor will give you a piece of candy soaked in the "contaminant," a yeast solution (a benign fungus). Roll it around in your right hand until your palm and fingers are very sticky. Put the candy in the disposal area designated by the instructor.

4. Shake hands with student number 2 in your group. Student 2 shakes hands with student 3, and so on, until *all but the last person* in the group has had a handshake.

5. Take a sterile cotton swab or inoculating loop, dip the cotton or loop end in the nutrient broth in the test tube, then swab your right hand with it. Carefully open your agar plate and gently rub the loop or streak the swab across the surface of the agar. Do not press too hard. Roll the tip as you streak to transfer as much of the material gathered from your hand as possible to the agar. Swab in a zigzag pattern as shown in Figure 2.3. Place the swab or loop in the area designated for disposal or clean-up.

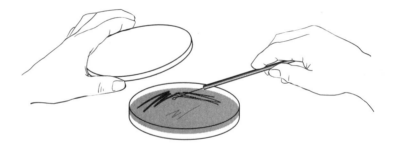

Figure 2.3
Streaking a plate

6. Cover the agar plate, turn it upside down (that is, agar side up), and store it at room temperature (approximately 25°C) to incubate for 24 hours.

7. Wash your hands thoroughly, then rinse with a dilute solution of disinfectant, if available.

8. **STOP & THINK** In your notebook, write a prediction of the results of this investigation.

9. After 24 hours of incubation, examine your plate and those of others in your group. Record whether or not there is growth on each of the plates.

▶ ANALYSIS

Write responses to the following questions in your notebook.

1. Which plate or plates have the most growth? The least? Make a chart showing the range of growth on plates from your group.

2. Did the results agree with your prediction? If not, why do you think they differed?

3. Why was the last person in your group instructed not to shake hands with anyone? How is that person's plate different from the others?

4. What might these results tell you about the spread of infectious disease?

5. What approaches can you think of to stop the spread of this classroom infection? Design an experiment that would prove that one of these approaches has stopped the spread. In your design be sure to include:
   – the question(s) being asked;
   – the hypothesis;
   – your predictions about the experimental results;
   – the experimental procedure you would use;
   – the method for data collection.

6. What might your experiment tell you about the possibility of reducing disease transmission in everyday life?

7. Do you think there is a danger in shaking hands with someone with smallpox? cholera? malaria? cancer? a genetic disease such as cystic fibrosis? Why or why not?

8. Read the article "U. S. Cholera Cases Set Record in 1992" on the following page. Based on the article and your knowledge, why do you think the admonition to "boil it, cook it, peel it or forget it" is good advice?

9. How might an airline learn more about infectious diseases that might be present in their route countries? What precautions might the airline take if they knew that cholera was present?

U.S. Cholera Cases Set Record in 1992

OUTBREAK FROM SINGLE FLIGHT ACCOUNTED FOR 75 OF 96 INCIDENTS OF ILLNESS

New York Times, September 11, 1992

ATLANTA, Sept. 10 (AP)—A cholera outbreak aboard an Argentine airplane bound for Los Angeles helped push the number of travel-related cholera cases in the United States to an all-time high, Federal health officials said today.

The airplane cases resulted from a cholera outbreak that began in Peru in 1991 and has now spread to Mexico and the Caribbean, resulting in 5,000 deaths along the way, the Federal Centers for Disease Control reported.

Cholera is a severe diarrhea that can be accompanied by vomiting and dehydration. It is caused by contaminated foods and water, and can be fatal in cases of extreme dehydration. The centers said that 96 cholera cases had been reported in the United States since January and that 95 of those were travel related. The cause of the remaining case is unknown.

OUTBREAK FROM FLIGHT

The number of cases this year is higher than in any year since the Federal agency began monitoring cholera in 1961. In the 20 years through 1981, only 10 cholera cases were reported in the United States, the agency reported.

The bulk of this year's cases resulted in February from a cholera outbreak aboard an Aerolineas Argentinas flight from Argentina to Los Angeles. Seventy-five passengers developed cholera from a seafood salad served during the flight. Most of the remaining cases involved Americans traveling to Latin America or Asia to visit relatives, the agency reported.

Travelers should avoid drinking water that has not been boiled and avoid eating raw seafood, raw vegetables and food or drinks sold by street vendors, said Dr. Jessica Tuttle, a medical epidemiologist for the centers. She said the agency recommended that travelers follow a general rule of "boil it, cook it, peel it or forget it."

The centers also recommended that airlines traveling to and from cholera-affected areas be equipped with special medicine to treat cholera patients.

The agency also reported today that the 1991 cholera outbreak in Latin America had now spread to Mexico and the Caribbean. More than 600,000 cholera cases and 5,000 deaths have been attributed to the outbreak through Aug. 26, the centers said. . .

EXTENDING IDEAS

- Analyze why and how prevention measures do or do not work. Trace the history of the treatment and prevention of diseases such as: measles, bubonic plague, hepatitis, diphtheria, the common cold, polio, smallpox, rabies, Lyme disease, herpes, tuberculosis, malaria, influenza, or AIDS and explain why methods of stopping the spread of the diseases succeeded or failed.

- The bubonic plague, or Black Death, originated in the Far East and spread west to Europe during the 1300s through shipping trade routes. These ships brought plague-ridden rats and infected seafarers to seaport cities. The symptoms of the plague included swelling of the lymph glands, pain, fever, and coughing up of blood. All of these preceded a painful death. Affected cities were filled with the unbearable stench exuding from bodies of the dead and dying. The nursery rhyme

    Ring a ring of rosies, a pocket full of posies
    A-tichoo, a-tichoo, we all fall down

    describes some of the symptoms and treatments of the time. Determine the trade routes during this period of time and how the path of the pandemic followed these routes. Explain how conditions during this time facilitated the spread of the disease, the nature of the treatments available to people, and what finally ended the pandemic.

- The course of history has been shaped by the occurrence of disease. Smallpox facilitated the Spanish conquest of America; Charlemagne's conquest of Europe in 876 A.D. was slowed by an epidemic of influenza which claimed much of his army; schistosomiasis is one of the reasons Taiwan is not part of mainland China today. Research one of these or other epidemics that have played a role in historical events.

- Are family pets factors in the transmission of diseases to humans? Is this a significant route of disease transmission? What precautions, if any, should pet owners take? Analyze local, regional, or state statistics to help answer the questions.

- Public health is a field that addresses the problem of disease prevention by studying conditions of environment, culture, and society that affect the health of a group of people. Call your nearest state public health office and interview a public health officer about his or her job.

PUBLIC HEALTH MICROBIOLOGIST   Does the seemingly invisible world which appears under a microscope fascinate you? Public health microbiologists are scientists who study microscopic life and the role of bacteria which cause disease by affecting the water or food supply or the general environment. They identify ways to control or eliminate sources of possible pollution or contagion. Microbiologists investigate disease-causing organisms in order to learn how the organism causes the disease. A microbiologist might count bacteria in a water supply and analyze sewage samples for harmful microorganisms. The laboratory techniques and procedures used by a microbiologist are not unique to microbiology, but are the techniques and equipment of chemists, geneticists, ecologists, or physiologists. With a four year college degree, positions as laboratory assistants, clinical or research microbiologists are possible. With a master's degree or doctoral degree, microbiologists can teach in a university or pursue independent research. Classes such as biology, chemistry, physics, mathematics, computer science, and English are necessary.

PUBLIC HEALTH SERVICE OFFICER   Are you interested in advocating for public health standards in your community? Public health service officers work with local communities, cities, states and federal or other authorities to advocate for the public health safety of a county or city. They may inspect facilities to ensure that public health standards are maintained, or to identify health hazards, assist in establishing clinics or other programs to improve public health, as well as to develop and coordinate public relations campaigns in order to promote services and programs within a community. They may also impose quarantines on specific areas, animals or persons known to be carrying contagious diseases, or prohibit the sale of unsafe food products or close establishments not meeting public health standards. Public health service officers have a four year college degree. Classes such as biology, chemistry, mathematics, computer science, and English are recommended.

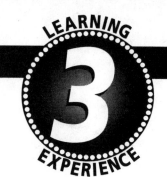

AGENTS OF DISEASE

PROLOGUE   Long before microbes were identified as the causative agents of infectious disease, humans pondered the origins of disease and of the devastating epidemics that often decimated human populations. In trying to find a reason for this suffering, different cultures developed various explanations for disease: unknown poisons, bad air, evil spirits, divine retribution. Disease was often viewed as divine punishment for sins or aberrant behavior, and afflicted individuals were tortured or even executed.

Even without any knowledge of microorganisms, careful observation of patterns of disease led groups of people to understand that certain diseases were *communicable* (spread by contact with other humans or animals and through food and water), and that they could be prevented by good hygiene and careful food preparation practices. But, what exactly was being communicated and causing disease?

In this learning experience, you will explore the agents that cause disease. Using your prior knowledge about the spread of disease and adding new information about the causative agents, you will determine what is causing sickness and death among young adults in New Mexico. Like epidemiologists, you will examine data, apply your understanding, and finally determine if there is a way to prevent the transmission of the disease.

BACTERIA AND VIRUSES AND PARASITES, OH MY!

Research in the late 1800s by a number of scientists provided evidence that many diseases were caused by microorganisms. The first conclusive demonstration that bacteria could cause disease was described in the work of Louis Pasteur and Robert Koch. Working independently, each scientist demonstrated that anthrax, a serious disease in domestic animals which is also transmissible to man, was caused by bacteria found in the bloodstream. The work of Pasteur, Koch, and other scientists in the field ushered in an era of discovery in which bacteria, viruses, and parasites were shown to be the causes of infectious diseases around the world.

In 1876, Koch proposed a set of criteria by which a microorganism could be determined to be an infectious agent (or *pathogen*). These criteria included:

- The microorganism must be present when the disease is present but absent in healthy organisms.
- It must be possible to isolate the microorganism.
- The isolated microorganism must cause disease when placed into a healthy organism.
- It must be possible to reisolate the microorganism from the second diseased host.

These criteria, called *Koch's Postulates*, are still used today to determine whether a disease is caused by an infectious agent. All organisms live in some kind of environment that provides them with nutrients and shelter in which to grow and replicate. In some cases, an infectious agent can survive in a number of different environments such as soil, water, a plant, or an animal, and it is only a matter of chance where the agent finally appears. In other cases, an infectious agent, for one reason or another, can live only within another organism, the host. Often the reason for this is that these pathogens require the nutrients that the host organism provides. The host becomes the environment from which the infectious agent derives everything it needs to survive. These organisms can only survive in one specific environment, which may be a plant or an animal or a bacterium. In some cases, the specificity may even extend to the type of tissue or cell in which the pathogen must live.

Wherever it lives, an infectious agent must grow and replicate. In order to do this, it must locate a suitable environment, take up nutrients, and release byproducts of its own metabolism. In carrying out these processes of life, the organism may deplete the nutrients in the environment, release toxic substances, and cause physical damage to its surroundings. The depletion of nutrients, damage from toxic substances, and mechanical damage can all contribute to causing the symptoms characteristic of the host's disease associated with that infectious agent. There are three major types of *pathogenic* (disease-causing) agents: bacteria, viruses, and parasites. Although fungi are also important in some diseases, they will not be considered here.

THE OLDEST ORGANISMS

For the first two billion years of Earth's existence, bacteria were its only tenants. Structurally the simplest of life forms, bacteria are single-celled prokaryotic organisms. Although capable of carrying out all of the cellular life functions, bacteria lack the internal structures, such as a nucleus and mitochondria, that are found in eukaryotic cells. Bacteria are also characterized by a cell wall, made up of polysaccharides, surrounding the cell membrane.

Bacteria constitute a large and diversified group of organisms. Capable of growing in a remarkably wide range of habitats and conditions, bacteria can be found just about anywhere—in the saltiest sea, in the hottest hot spring, and in the most acid or alkaline conditions. They make the soil fertile: in every gram of fertile soil there exist about 100,000,000 living bacteria; this amounts to about 90–250 kg (200–550 lb) of bacteria for every acre of soil. Bacteria decompose dead organic matter, help plants obtain vital nitrogen from the air, help us make vitamins and fend off undesirable microbes, and provide us with some of life's pleasures, such as yogurt and cheese. Most mammals are walking apartment complexes for a wide variety of bacteria, some of which are essential to the well-being of the animal, most of which are just along for the ride.

Despite their abundance and diversity of species, bacteria are remarkably lacking in variety when it comes to shape and distinguishing structural features. They can be spherical, as are the bacteria *Streptococcus pyogenes* (the causative agent of sore throats); rod-shaped, as are *Salmonella typhi* (the cause of

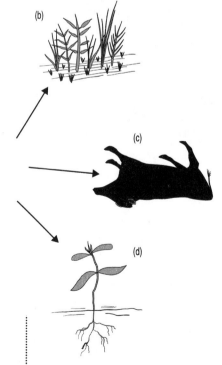

Figure 3.1
Bacteria carry out many roles in life: (a) helping animals make vitamins; (b) keeping the soil fertile; (c) decomposing dead matter; (d) fixing nitrogen into nitrates; (e) carrying out processes that result in cheese.

typhoid fever), *Vibrio cholerae* (the causative agent of cholera), and *Pseudomonas aeruginosa* (bacteria commonly found in soil); or they can be helical or spiral-shaped, as are *Treponema pallidum* (the cause of syphilis) and *Spirochaeta picatilis* (large and harmless spirochete common in water).

Because bacteria have limited mobility, they must rely on carriers such as animals, water, or food. Insect bites and fecal material from birds, rodents, cats and other animals can also transmit bacteria. Though most people are scarcely aware of the bacteria around them, life would be very difficult—if not impossible—without bacteria. Despite all the important things bacteria provide, people generally only recognize the existence of bacteria when they become ill. For this reason, bacteria are generally viewed as "bad." Like all living things, however, bacteria are only carrying out the processes of life, which include taking nutrients from their environment so that they can grow and reproduce. For the majority of bacteria, this environment is the soil or water, but for others, this environment is another organism. That organism may become diseased as a result.

The troublesome, pathogenic bacteria are only a small portion of the total bacterial world. Lewis Thomas in "On Disease" put it this way:

> *It is true, of course, that germs are all around us; they comprise a fair proportion of the sheer bulk of the soil, and they abound in the air. But it is certainly not true that they are our natural enemies. Indeed, it comes as a surprise to realize that such a tiny minority of the bacterial populations of the earth has any interest at all in us. . . It is probably true that symbiotic relationships between bacteria and their . . . hosts are much more common in nature than infectious disease. . . . But if you count up all the indispensable microbes that live in various intestinal tracts, supplying essential nutrients or providing enzymes for the breakdown of otherwise indigestible food, and add all the peculiar bacterial aggregates that live like necessary organs in the tissues of many insects, plus all the bacterial symbionts engaged in nitrogen fixation in collaboration with legumes, the total mass of symbiotic life is overwhelming. Alongside, the list of important bacterial infections of human beings is short indeed.*

> *Excerpted from "On Disease," copyright (c) 1979 by Lewis Thomas, from* The Medusa and the Snail *by Lewis Thomas. used by permission of Viking Penguin, a division of Penguin Books USA, Inc.*

When bacteria do cause disease they can do it in a variety of ways. Living in blood, on skin, on mucous membranes, and sometimes within

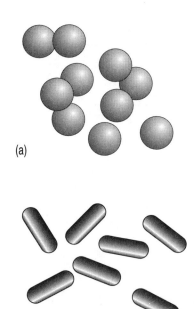

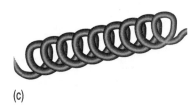

Figure 3.2
Three shapes of bacteria: (a) spherical; (b) rod-shaped; (c) helical.

(a)

(b)

(c)

cells, these tiny invaders may secrete toxic substances that damage vital tissues, feast on nutrients intended for the cell, or may form colonies that disrupt normal functions in the host's body. Directly or indirectly, their actions can cause extensive damage to the host.

The presence of bacterial cell walls makes some bacteria susceptible to treatment with antibiotics. *Antibiotics* are chemical compounds that either kill or inhibit the growth of bacteria. Certain antibiotics act by interfering with the synthesis of the cell wall. Because animal cells do not have a cell wall, antibiotics affect only the infecting bacteria. When first discovered in the 1920s, antibiotics were viewed as miracle drugs capable of saving humankind from the devastating diseases that had plagued them throughout history. However, almost as soon as a new antibiotic was discovered, certain bacteria with the ability to resist its killing effect were found. These were able to survive and multiply while the more susceptible bacteria were killed. Bacterial resistance to antibiotics is now one of the biggest challenges facing medical practitioners today.

THE VIRAL INVADER

Viruses have an enormous impact on human beings and, like bacteria, have been part of our lives since at least the beginning of recorded time. A *bas relief* from 1500 B.C. Egypt depicts a priest with a shriveled leg, evidence of infection with polio virus. A thirteenth-century manuscript shows a dog, mouth foaming, attacking a terrified man destined to die from the rabies virus transmitted from a dog bite. Smallpox is believed to have helped a small band of Spaniards under Cortés subdue the vast and powerful Aztec nation.

These microbes, too small to be visible even under the light microscope, were discovered not long after bacteria were implicated as the causative agent in anthrax. Their existence was demonstrated in 1892 by the Russian scientist Dimitri Ivanovsky, who was investigating the cause of a disease in tobacco plants.

As perpetrators of disease, viruses have been viewed as one of the "bad guys" of the microbial world. Variously termed "pirates of the cell", "viral hitchhikers", "cellular hijackers", and "pieces of bad news wrapped up in protein", these tiny microbes have been perceived as having evil intent. In reality, viruses are just simple microbes, genetic material (that is, nucleic acid) surrounded by protein. A virus is not a cell. It cannot maintain the characteristics of life on its own. Lacking the biochemical and structural components (cellular machinery) that enable an organism to carry out the life processes—no membrane, no nucleus, no mitochondria and thus no capacity to take up and utilize nutrients—it cannot reproduce, metabolize, or conduct any of the basic processes of life. A virus must seek out an environment that provides not only the nutrients it needs to carry out life processes but also the cellular machinery required for these processes—that is, a cell. A virus cannot live outside a cell. Viruses exist for almost every kind of cell: bacterial, plant, fungal, and animal.

Much smaller than any cell, a typical virus is comprised of a protein "coat" surrounding its viral genetic material (see Figure 3.3). This genetic material contains specific instructions for making identical copies of the virus. The proteins encoded by the viral genes must be able to take over the cellular machinery of the cell; this "commandeered machinery" is then used to aid the reproduction of the virus and, in many cases, is no longer available for the growth and reproduction of the invaded cell. A virus enters the cell and, using different mechanisms depending on the kind of virus it is, causes the cell to stop making what it needs for itself and instead makes what the virus needs to reproduce. Like an unwanted guest who eats everything in the refrigerator, uses every clean towel in the house, and on leaving reduces your house to a pile of rubble, the virus utilizes the building blocks and energy stored that the cell has generated for its own growth and reproduction. The cell is depleted of the materials and energy it needs to repair the damage. The machinery the cell needs to make more of itself is no longer under its control. As a result, the cell often dies from this invasion.

Having no cell walls, viruses are not susceptible to antibiotics. Unlike the discovery of antibiotics for treating bacteria, no "miracle" drugs have been discovered for the treatment of viruses. In fact, to date, no truly effective *viricidal* (virus killing) drugs

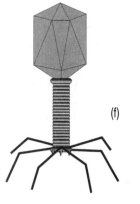

(a)

(b)

(c)

(d)

(e)

(f)

Figure 3.3
Various kinds of viruses: (a) tobacco mosaic virus; (b) human immunodeficiency virus (HIV); (c) polio virus; (d) Ebola virus; (e) influenza virus; (f) bacteriophage T4.

exist. In most instances, treatment of viral infections involves prevention (vaccines) or in helping the body to help itself, which means sleeping, drinking plenty of fluids, and eating chicken soup.

THE PARASITIC WAY OF LIFE

The parasitic way of life is highly successful. There are far more kinds of parasitic than nonparasitic organisms in the world. Those organisms which are not parasites are usually hosts. Even parasites are often hosts for other parasites. Or, in the words of Jonathan Swift:

> *Big fleas have little fleas*
> *upon their backs to bite 'em,*
> *Little fleas have lesser fleas and so,* ad infinitum

The parasitic way of life is one form of living relationship called *symbiosis*. A symbiotic relationship involves any two organisms that live together in close association, often with mutually beneficial results and sometimes not. When a symbiont actually lives at the expense of the host, that is, uses nutrients required by the host, then it is called a *parasite*. Some parasites live their entire mature lives within or on the host, but others, such as fleas or mosquitoes, only visit for a meal—they eat and run (or fly). Parasites can be unicellular protozoa, such as the plasmodia that live inside red blood cells and are the causative agent of malaria, the major infectious disease in the world today; worms such as tapeworms, which live in the digestive tract; schistosomes that inhabit the veins of the bladder or intestines and are the causative agents of schistosomiasis; or arthropods, such as fleas and ticks, temporary parasites that visit the host for frequent or occasional feedings. There are also parasitic fungi, including mushrooms, molds, and mildews which feed on plants or animals. By this definition, certain bacteria and viruses can be considered to live as parasites. In the conventional definition, the term parasite refers only to eukaryotic organisms.

A parasite is often associated with damage to the host. A parasite may harm its host in any of a number of ways: by mechanical injury, such as boring a hole in it; by eating or digesting and absorbing its tissues; by poisoning the host with toxic metabolic products; or simply by robbing the host of nutrients. Most parasites inflict a combination of these conditions on their hosts. Of

Figure 3.4
Various kinds of parasites: (a) plasmodia, microscopic parasites in a red blood cell; (b) tapeworm, a flatworm that can grow to more than 10 M in length; (c) tick, an insect the size of a pinhead. (Pictures not drawn to scale.)

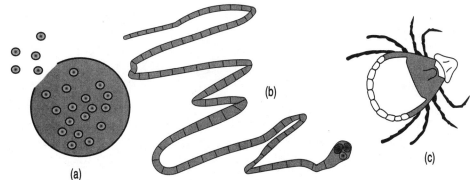

(a)   (b)   (c)

course, the parasite is only trying to survive, taking from its environment what it needs to sustain its life processes so that it can reproduce. Parasites do not have evil intent, any more than bacteria or viruses do.

The treatment of parasitic diseases reflects the great diversity of parasites. Many unicellular parasites can be treated with drugs such as quinine for malaria and arsenic derivatives for sleeping sickness. Tapeworms and nematodes can also be treated with drugs which interfere with their metabolism. Although no vaccines exist to date, many parasitic diseases can be prevented by good hygiene, sanitary facilities, and effective programs of insect control. A simple change of habits, such as staying out of lakes and rivers, could prevent many serious, debilitating diseases. Parasites can be transmitted in a variety of ways: in contaminated food or water, by direct contact, or in the feces or saliva of an insect or other animal.

THE HOST-INFECTIOUS AGENT INTERACTION

Despite their great diversity in structure and habits, all infectious agents have the same life requirements for survival: to grow and to reproduce themselves. These requirements, in fact, are shared with all living things. To fulfill these needs all living things must obtain nutrients and live at appropriate temperatures and levels of moisture, pH and oxygen. Organisms derive these essential components from their environment, which in the case of infectious agents, happens to be another living organism.

In many instances, the organism in which the infectious agent has taken up residence is not always a gracious host. Many host organisms have evolved ways to try to rid themselves of unwanted houseguests. Animals, plants, and even bacteria have developed a wide arsenal of physical, chemical, and biological strategies against invading organisms. In humans, the immune system has developed an elegant and complex response to infectious agents. Specific proteins called *antibodies* are made in response to almost every foreign substance that enters the body. (In fact, invading organisms can often be identified based on the kind of antibodies present in the body.) These antibodies bind to the foreign substance and mark it for destruction. If this substance is part of a virus, bacteria, or parasite, the organism may be doomed.

Antibodies are one kind of host response against infection; specialized cells are another. Certain cells of the immune system are mobilized and become an army of white blood cells that circulate through the body and destroy the invaders. The function of these white blood cells is to engulf and destroy pathogens, and to produce toxic substances designed to kill infected cells and invading organisms.

As with all living things, infectious organisms affect their environment as they grow. It does not benefit the infectious agent to harm its environment in the process of living, since the well-being of that environment or host is essential to the infectious agent's own well-being. Many host–infectious agent relationships exist in a balance in which the two partners have evolved to tolerance; the agent takes from the host what it needs without damaging the host, and the host tolerates the presence of the agent by not defending itself too vigorously. Other host–infectious agent relationships have not reached this level of tolerance, and the result is disease.

▶ ANALYSIS

1. How would you define an infectious disease? A noninfectious disease?

2. What is meant when an organism is termed an "infectious agent"?

3. Create a table that compares each type of infectious agent— bacterium, virus, and parasite—using the following criteria:
   a. how the agent is spread
   b. the symptoms this agent might cause
   c. biological characteristics of this agent and the significance of its characteristics
   d. methods of treatment

4. Why do some infectious agents make you sick?

THE CASE OF THE KILLER CONGESTION

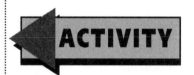

INTRODUCTION

*L*ong-distance runner Merrill Bahe was on his way to his girlfriend's funeral on May 14, 1993, when he found himself gasping for air. Suddenly, and quite dramatically, Bahe was overcome with fever, headache, and respiratory distress. In the presence of his grief-stricken relatives, Bahe gulped desperately for air in their car, en route south to Gallup, New Mexico.

Minutes later the nineteen-year-old Navajo athlete was dead.

His twenty-four-year old girlfriend had died in a small Indian Health Service clinic located sixty miles away from Gallup a few days earlier after an identical bout of sudden respiratory illness. And within the week her brother and his girl-

friend, also young, athletic Navajos, who lived in trailers near
Bahe's, fell mysteriously ill; the young woman died.

Excerpt from The Coming Plague *by*
Laurie Garrett, copyright 1994.
Reprinted by permission of Farrar,
Straus and Giroux, Inc., page 528.

Chilled by the sudden deaths of these apparently healthy, young adults, attending physician Bruce Tempest put out a call to other physicians and colleagues in the state, describing the symptoms and requesting immediate notification if other cases were seen. By the end of the day he had compiled a list of five more healthy young people who had died of acute respiratory distress syndrome. Within the week the list grew to nineteen suspected cases, twelve of whom had died.

The disease seemed to follow the same pattern in every victim. It started with flu-like symptoms of fever, muscle aches, and headaches. After a period of a few hours to two days, those symptoms worsened to coughing and irritation in the lungs which seemed to be caused by leaks in the capillary network feeding the lungs with blood. This leakage of the plasma fluid from the blood filled the air sacs of the lungs. Shortly thereafter, the patients were unable to absorb oxygen from the air they took into their lungs. Starving for oxygen, the heart would slow down and death could soon follow.

▶ **TASK**

As a modern epidemiologist would, you must determine what is causing the killer respiratory distress syndrome, how it is being transmitted, and then determine if anything can be done to stop the epidemic. Like teams of epidemiologists from the Centers for Disease Control and Prevention (CDC), your group will familiarize yourselves with information about the characteristics of a wide range of diseases and with the data about the specific epidemic.

When researching epidemics, time is always of the essence. The disease continues to spread. The longer you take to solve the problem the more deaths occur. You will have more than enough information so you must think carefully about the data, identify which data gives you information that will help you determine the causative agent, and determine which data is still inconclusive.

Each team will need to complete a report that records the decisions and information that led you to the identification of the causative agent and outlines your solutions to stopping the epidemic. For your report, you will need to do the following:

- Read the epidemiological, medical, and laboratory reports that follow.

- Examine Table 3.5, "Causes of Respiratory Distress," which contains information about various causes of respiratory distress and hemorrhagic (bleeding) symptoms and their characteristics.

- Use each report and your table to eliminate candidates.

- Record your rationale for each decision. For example, record how you decided whether the disease was infectious or noninfectious.

- Use the table you created from the Analysis of "Bacteria and Viruses and Parasites, Oh My!" to ensure that you have a complete picture.

- Write a report that contains the following information:
  - The nature of the epidemic; is it an infectious or noninfectious disease?
  - The probable causative agent of the epidemic, if infectious.
  - The process by which you came to the decision about the causative agent.
  - Diagnostic procedures to use on a new patient demonstrating symptoms of the disease.
  - Potential treatment for the disease.
  - The rationale for each decision.
  - Recommendations for preventing further spread of the disease.

- Be prepared to present the results of the data and your recommendations for stopping the epidemic to your fellow epidemiological teams.

REPORT ONE: EPIDEMIOLOGICAL DATA

1. Data about infected individuals (victims)

   Geographical distribution—lived in New Mexico and other parts of the Southwest, South, and Northwest United States

   Habits—worked in a variety of jobs; some held positions in maintenance or cleaning; no unusual hobbies

   Living Conditions—lived in trailers, small homes; generally in rural areas

   Relationships—in some cases victims were related; one instance of engaged couple as victims; primarily isolated cases of unrelated, uninvolved individuals

   Travel—no pattern of foreign travel or association with anyone who has traveled

2. Data about environment

   Recent rains and good growing conditions for seeds, nuts, berries, and insects had resulted in increase in rodent population.

REPORT TWO: MEDICAL DATA

1. *Symptoms*—respiratory distress, flu-like symptoms, fever, muscle aches, coughing, difficulty in obtaining oxygen

2. *Victims*—range of ages; many young adults

3. *Treatment*—antibiotics ineffective; no response to anti-protozoal drugs (drugs which eliminate parasitic, single-celled organisms or protozoans)

4. *Autopsy report*:
   - death by suffocation
   - rapid occurrence of death after onset of symptoms
   - air sacs in lungs filled with fluid, presumably from blood plasma leaking from pulmonary (lung) veins

REPORT THREE: LABORATORY DATA

1. *Mass spectral analysis*—negative for chemical toxins and heavy metals

2. *Examination of lung tissue and blood smears by direct stain and light microscopic analysis*—negative for visible pathogens

3. *Growth in culture from blood and lung tissue*—no growth demonstrated

4. *Immunology Report*:
   - large increase in number of white blood cells
   - results of antibody detection assays:
     - negative for *Toxoplasma gondii, Streptococcus pneumoniae, Mycoplasma*, influenza virus
     - inconclusive for Ebola virus, hantavirus, pneumocystis, Legionella, *Pasteurella pestis*

Table 3.5

Causes of Respiratory Distress	Type of Agent	Mode of Transmission	Geographic Location	Symptoms	Main Target Population	Treatment	Nature of Immune Response	Location in Body	Method of Detection	Prognosis
phosgene	chemical toxin; poison gas	aerosol as gas	worldwide	coughing; fluid filled lungs	all ages	NA*	NA*	blood; lungs; other tissues	mass spectral analysis**	damage to lungs
paraquat	chemical toxin; herbicide	ingestion of treated plants	South America; Central America	cough; congestion; fluid filled lungs	all ages	NA*	NA*	blood; lungs; renal and skeletal tissue	mass spectral analysis**	damage to lungs
influenza	virus	airborne; human to human	worldwide	fever; cough; muscle pain	all ages	bedrest; fluids	white blood cells; antibodies	inside a cell; lungs	antibody detection***	death in elderly and sickly; otherwise recovery
Ebola	virus	direct contact; human to human	Africa	internal bleeding; fluid loss	all ages	bedrest; fluids	white blood cells; antibodies	inside a cell; blood vessels	antibody detection***	80% death rate
hantavirus	virus	airborne; aerosol of mice feces	Asia; U.S.	congestion; fever; fluid filled lungs	all ages; especially adults between 20 and 60	bedrest; fluids	white blood cells; antibodies	inside a cell; blood vessels in lungs	antibody detection***	70% death rate
plague	bacteria (*Pasteurella pestis*)	fleas living on rodents	worldwide	fever; swollen lymphs; cough; pain	all ages	antibiotics	antibodies	lungs; blood; lymph glands	direct stain of blood smears; antibody detection***; culture****	generally fatal if untreated
Legionnaires' disease	bacteria (*Legionella*)	aerosol; "scum water" from appliances	U.S.	fever; muscle aches; congestion	all ages; older adults	antibiotics (often resistant)	antibodies	lungs; blood	direct stain of blood smears; antibody detection***; difficult to culture****	can be fatal if untreated

Continued on next page

CAUSES OF RESPIRATORY DISTRESS	TYPE OF AGENT	MODE OF TRANSMISSION	GEOGRAPHIC LOCATION	SYMPTOMS	MAIN TARGET POPULATION	TREATMENT	NATURE OF IMMUNE RESPONSE	LOCATION IN BODY	METHOD OF DETECTION	PROGNOSIS
Mycoplasma pneumonia	bacteria	airborne; human to human	worldwide	persistent cough; fever; congestion	all ages	antibiotics	white blood cells; antibodies	inside a cell; lungs	antibody detection***; difficult to culture****	generally complete recovery
bacterial pneumonia (*Streptococcus* pneumonia)	bacteria	airborne; human to human	worldwide	cough; fever; ear ache	children	antibiotics (often resistant)	antibodies	connective tissue; lungs; ear canals	antibody detection***; culture****	generally complete recovery; may persist
Toxoplasma	parasitic protozoan	cat feces; undercooked meat	worldwide	congestion; convulsion paralysis; heart disease	newborns; generally asymptomatic in adults	anti-protozoal drugs	white blood cells; antibodies	inside a cell; lungs	antibody detection***	eventual recovery; may cause birth defects
Pneumocystic pneumonia	parasitic protozoan	believed to be airborne; human to human	Europe; U.S.	high fever in adults; air sacs filled with foam	malnourished children; weakened adults	anti-protozoal drugs	white blood cells; antibodies	inside a cell; lungs	direct stain of sputum; antibody detection***	often fatal

Notes for Table:

*   NA means that the information is not available.

**   mass spectral analysis is an assay for detecting chemical substances and heavy metals in blood and tissue.

***   Antibody detection is an assay in which the blood of victims is mixed with purified infectious agents. If antibodies specific to those organisms are present in the blood of victims, clumping will be seen in the sample, indicating that the antibody has bound to the added microorganism and that the person is most likely infected with that microorganism.

**** Culture is the growth of the organism on agar as you did in Learning Experience 2.

EXTENDING IDEAS

Long before the demonstration that microbes were responsible for disease and that these pathogens could be transmitted via water, food, air and animals, many cultures had established rituals, taboos, and customs which, in part, were developed to avoid illnesses observed to be associated with certain hygienic or food practices. The Navajo had long ago made a connection between mice and disease, as evidenced by the following excerpt from "Death at the Corners."

When a mysterious mouse-borne illness began claiming the lives of young Navajos last spring, tribal elders blamed the deaths on the tendency of young generations to drift away from traditional belief. The elders may have been right.

Contact with mice has always been prohibited in Navajo culture. While mice are revered because they brought life to the world by spreading seeds, they are also thought to have dangerous powers. They belong to the night world, whereas humans belong to the day world, and the two must remain apart. Mice must be kept out of houses and away from food, and if a mouse so much as touches your clothes, the garments must be burned...

From a medicine woman in Monument Valley, Muneta [a doctor from the Indian Health Service] learned that mice must never be touched or allowed in the home because they are "bearers of illness from ancient times." Their droppings and saliva are believed to cause disease. Anything a mouse touches might be contaminated, hence the requirement to burn clothing. The Navajo word for mouse, na'atoosi, *means "the one that sucks on things." The implication, says Muneta, is that it leaves behind its saliva . . .*

Muneta translated the mouse's power into the aerosolized viral particles [from the mouse droppings] that spread disease. She [the medicine woman] also told him that "the mouse would choose the strongest and best person in the house." Unlike other infectious ailments, hantaviral diseases tend to strike young healthy adults rather than small children and the elderly.

> *Excerpted from "The Mouse Injunction" from Death at the Corners by Denise Grady,* Discover Magazine, *December 1993, pp. 83–91.*

Describe a tradition, ritual, or custom that you think is based on an understanding of infectious disease and its spread. Provide a possible explanation of what kind of infectious disease it might have been designed to prevent and how this custom might achieve this.

Parasitic diseases in developing countries are a great drain on the economic infrastructures of these countries. Research one disease caused by a parasite. Then describe the parasite's life cycle, the symptoms of the disease, and how this disease could cause financial loss in the country.

ON THE JOB

EPIDEMIOLOGIST   Are you interested in solving problems, looking for clues or identifying patterns? Epidemiologists plan and conduct studies to examine trends in the incidence of disease and the public health impact of a specific disease. An environmental epidemiologist studies the incidence of disease in industrial areas and the effects of industrial chemicals on health. Epidemiologists plan and collect data such as areas in which disease is located, any relationships between victims, relevant medical data, known information about the cause of disease (viral, bacterial, genetic) and the mode of transmission. Next epidemiologists analyze data to identify possible causative agents and the mode of transmission to identify treatment and prevent further spreading of the disease. Epidemiologists may work in universities, for government organizations such as the Centers for Disease Control and Prevention (CDC) or for nonprofit organizations such as the American Cancer Society. Epidemiologists have a minimum four year college degree in biological or applied sciences and often a master's or doctorate from a school of public health. Classes such as biology, chemistry, epidemiology, mathematics, statistics, English,and computer science are recommended.

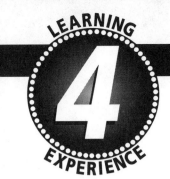

Search for the Cause

PROLOGUE   In the previous learning experience, you were introduced to different causative agents of disease. What makes these organisms pathogenic? What special characteristics make these organisms harmful to their hosts? Is one factor responsible for the virulence of all these organisms, or many different factors? These are some of the questions scientists ask as they investigate infectious diseases. In this learning experience, you will analyze an important experiment carried out in an attempt to answer these questions, and conduct an experiment that investigates the factor(s) responsible for virulence in organisms.

Griffith's Search for the Cause

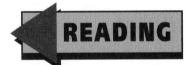

By the early 1900s, the notion that contagious diseases were the result of infectious agents had been accepted. From that time on, a major focus of research into infectious disease would be to understand the mechanisms by which these infectious agents caused the symptoms of disease in their hosts. In 1928, a British bacteriologist named Frederick Griffith was investigating the way in which a certain type of bacteria, *Diplococcus pneumoniae*, caused pneumonia, a serious and often fatal lung disease. Scientists already knew which type of bacteria caused the disease, but they were trying to learn how the bacteria caused the disease.

Griffith studied two strains of *D. pneumoniae*. Both grew very well in special culture media in his laboratory, but only one of them actually caused pneumonia when injected into mice. Griffith noticed that when he grew the bacteria on nutrient agar plates in the laboratory he could distinguish one strain from the other simply by its appearance on the agar. Each bacterium in the *virulent*, or disease-causing strain, secretes a polysaccharide (sugar) coat called a *capsule* around its cell wall. Bacteria grow in colonies (a discrete mass of cells) on agar, and colonies of the virulent strain look smooth because of their capsules. Though Griffith did not know it then, we now understand that the capsules protect the bacteria from destruction by the host animal's immune response, allowing them to multiply and grow in the host. The other, *nonvirulent* strain Griffith studied did not produce capsules. Instead, when grown on agar the colonies, it appeared to have rough, jagged edges. The lack of polysaccharide capsules made this strain vulnerable to the immune system; when it entered a host it was destroyed by the immune response and was, therefore, nonpathogenic. (see Figure 4.1)

disease causing ability	appearance of agar plate	diagram of colony appearance on agar plate
nonencapsulated bacteria (does not cause disease)	rough edged colonies	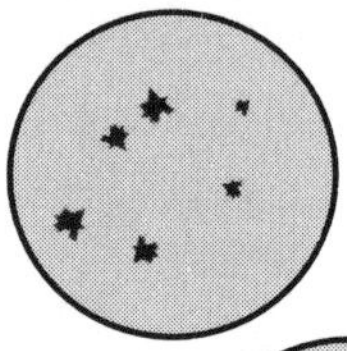
encapsulated bacteria (causes disease)	smooth colonies	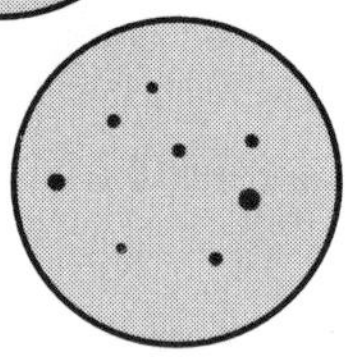

Figure 4.1
Summary of characteristics of the two strains of *D. pneumoniae*

Griffith hypothesized that the capsule might be responsible for the disease in some way. He had two important pieces of information (data) before he started the experiment: that the encapsulated bacteria could kill mice and that the nonencapsulated bacteria could not. With this information he was able to design a simple experiment providing a critical result, one that led investigators to the mechanisms by which these organisms can cause disease and acquire characteristics such as virulence. Figure 4.2 (on the next page) summarizes Griffith's experiments. Examine it and respond to the Analysis questions.

▶ ANALYSIS

1. What simple question did Griffith pose in this experiment?
2. What parts of the experiment represented the controls? Describe how these served as controls.
3. If Griffith believed that the polysaccharide capsule of the encapsulated strain was responsible for its disease-causing characteristic,

what do you think he predicted would be the results of injecting the heat-killed, encapsulated bacteria alone? Why?

4. Why do you think the mouse died when Griffith mixed and injected the dead, virulent strain with the live, nonvirulent strain?

5. If you could isolate the bacteria that were injected as live, nonvirulent bacteria in the last experiment, how could you determine whether they had changed characteristics and had become virulent?

Figure 4.2
Griffith's experiment

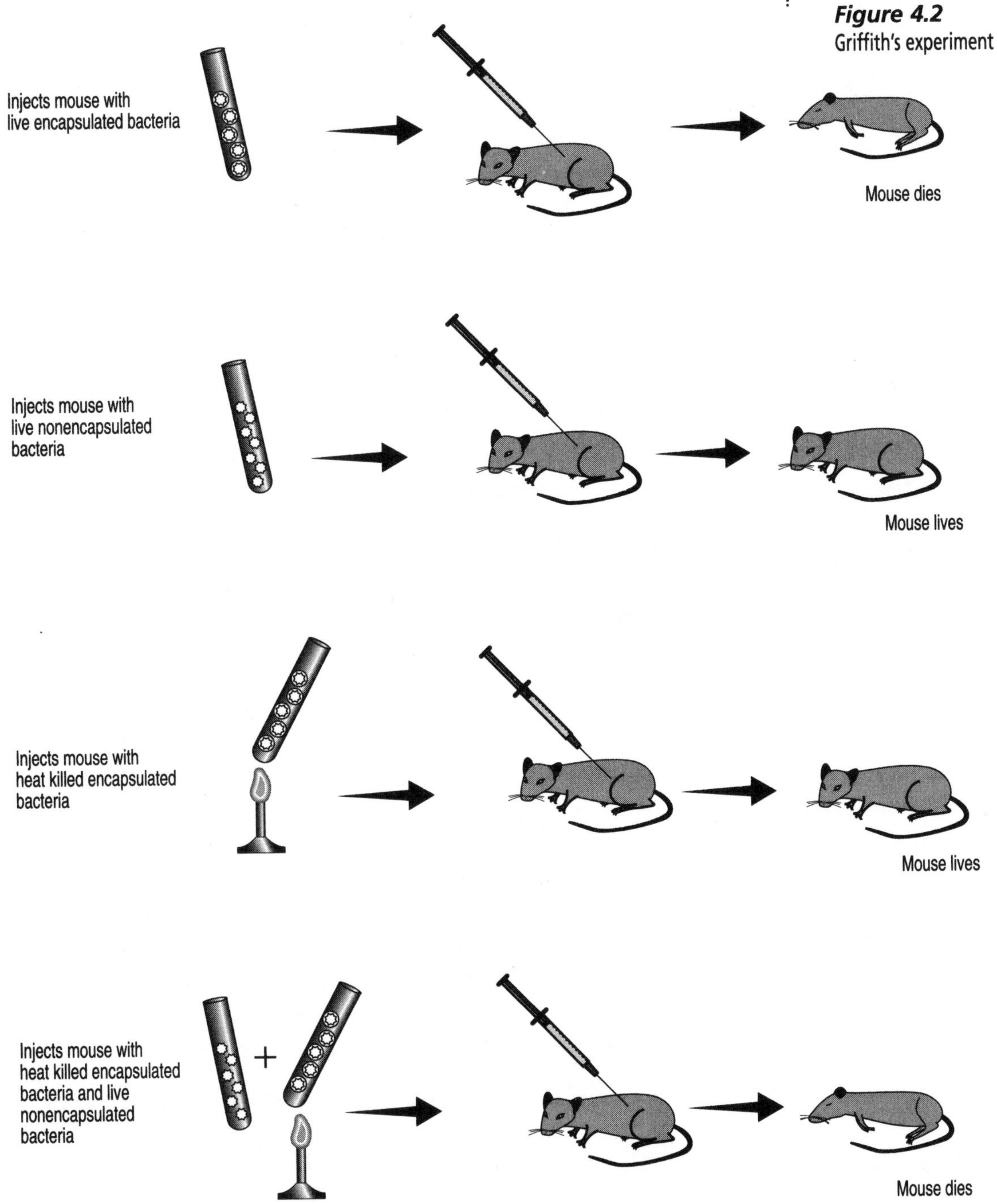

Injects mouse with live encapsulated bacteria

Mouse dies

Injects mouse with live nonencapsulated bacteria

Mouse lives

Injects mouse with heat killed encapsulated bacteria

Mouse lives

Injects mouse with heat killed encapsulated bacteria and live nonencapsulated bacteria

Mouse dies

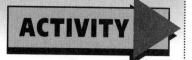

IN ISOLATION

INTRODUCTION   When Griffith reisolated the originally nonvirulent strain from the dead mice in his experiment, he observed that this strain no longer formed rough colonies on nutrient agar plates, but formed smooth colonies. When these were injected into mice, the mice died of pneumonia. Somehow the nonvirulent, nonencapsulated strain had been changed, or transformed, into the pathogenic, encapsulated strain. Some principle or factor had been transferred from the killed, virulent strain to the live, nonvirulent strain, giving it the ability to make a polysaccharide capsule and cause disease.

For more than 15 years afterward, researchers attempted to identify what had happened in Griffith's experiment. What had changed the harmless strain into a virulent form? In 1944, Oswald T. Avery, Colin MacLeod, and Maclyn McCarty took the extract from dead virulent bacteria and one by one removed the biomolecules of the cell—first the proteins, then the carbohydrates, next the lipids, leaving the nucleic acids—each time testing the ability of that substance to make nonvirulent bacteria virulent.

In the following laboratory experiment you will use a procedure similar to that used by Avery, MacLeod, and McCarty to isolate the factor that transformed the harmless strain of bacteria into a virulent form. In your isolation you will be working with thymus or liver tissue rather than with *D. pneumoniae*. The same principles that Avery and his colleagues used to isolate the transforming factor apply to any living organism. Thymus and liver are more readily available, not virulent, and easier to work with than bacteria.

Before carrying out the actual isolation experiment, read the entire procedure in order to determine the principles behind the experiment.

▶ MATERIALS NEEDED

For each pair of students:
- 2 pairs of safety goggles
- 1.0 mL of a homogenate of blended fresh thymus or liver (keep on ice)
- 2.0 mL salt (NaCl) solution
- 1 test tube (13 x 100 mm) with cap (or, cover with plastic wrap)

- 1 test tube rack (or small beaker to hold test tube)
- 5 mL ice-cold ethanol
- 1 glass stirring rod
- 1 ice water bath
- plastic wrap
- 2 10-mL conical centrifuge tubes with lids (optional)

For the class:
- 1 tabletop centrifuge (optional)

PROCEDURE

Use the Procedure Analysis column of Table 4.3, with the diagram of the cell that follows the table (Figure 4.4), in order to describe what is happening at the cellular level at each stage of the investigation. It is important to remember that these are the same principles Avery's team used when isolating the "transforming factor" from bacteria (they may have used different chemicals).

SAFETY NOTE: *Always wear safety goggles when conducting experiments.*

Table 4.3

PROCEDURE	PRINCIPLES INVOLVED	PROCEDURE ANALYSIS
1*. Blend together thymus with the buffer which contains: – sugar – aspirin – Epsom salts – water – detergent solution (*provided by teacher)	Detergent dissolves lipids and denatures proteins. Epsom salts and aspirin inactivate enzymes that degrade nucleic acid (DNA).	What does the detergent do to the cell? What parts of the cell are affected? Why are aspirin and Epsom salts added? What does the blending do?
2. Pour homogenate into a beaker. Place 1 mL in test tube or centrifuge tube. Add 2 mL of salt solution (NaCl and water) and shake well for two minutes.	Salt breaks up membranes further.	What effect is the salt having on the cell? Using the cell diagram, describe what has happened to the cell in steps 1 and 2.
3. If possible (this step is optional), spin tubes in a tabletop centrifuge for seven minutes. Be sure tubes are balanced. Remove tube from centrifuge and carefully pour off liquid into a clean test tube, being sure not to dislodge pellet.	High speed centrifugation separates larger structures such as membrane fragments from smaller, soluble biomolecules.	What is in the pellet? What is in the liquid?
4. Place test tube in an ice bath and leave for five minutes.	Cold temperatures slow down the action of enzymes.	Why is it advisable to keep the liquid cold?
5. Carefully pour or pipette 5 mL ice-cold ethanol down the side of the tube to form a layer on top of the water layer.	Nucleic acid is soluble in water but insoluble in ethanol.	What is happening when the ethanol is added?
6. Leave test tube undisturbed in ice water bath for 10 minutes.		

Continued on next page

PROCEDURE	PRINCIPLES INVOLVED	PROCEDURE ANALYSIS
7. After 10 minutes, dip the end of a glass stirring rod into the cell/ethanol mix. Slide the rod back and forth between the layers while spinning the rod with your fingertips.		
8. Place the material attached to the rod on a piece of plastic wrap. Roll it, stretch it, play with it.		What is the material on the glass rod?

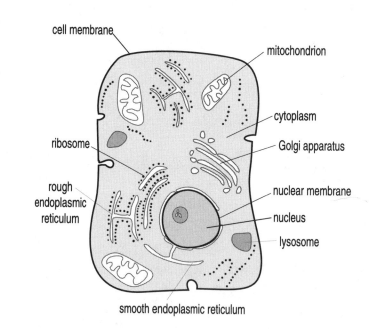

Figure 4.4
Parts of an animal cell as seen under a microscope.

Table 4.5

CELL PART	BIOMOLECULE COMPOSITION
cell membrane	lipid, protein
endoplasmic reticulum	lipid, protein, nucleic acid
ribosome	protein, nucleic acid
Golgi apparatus	lipid, protein
lysosome	lipid, protein
cytoplasm	lipid, protein, nucleic acid, carbohydrate
mitochondrion	lipid, protein, nucleic acid, carbohydrate
nuclear membrane	lipid, protein
nucleus	lipid, protein, nucleic acid

▶ ANALYSIS

1. In your notebook, diagram the components of a thymus or liver cell and indicate where the transforming material is located.

2. In a flow diagram, indicate what you think happens to the cell during the following stages of the procedure:
   - when adding the buffer solution and detergent;
   - when blending;
   - when adding the salt solution.

3. Describe why each biomolecule may or may not be a good candidate for the transforming property.

4. What is on your glass rod? Avery's team isolated this very same kind of material from the *D. pneumoniae* bacteria and determined that it was responsible for transforming the harmless bacteria. If what you have on your glass rod had been isolated from bacteria instead of thymus, how would you determine that this material was responsible for transforming the nonvirulent strain into the virulent strain? Design an experiment to show whether the harmless bacteria would be changed by this material.

5. Avery's team had isolated the material that could change an organism with one set of physical traits into an organism with a different set of physical traits. Explain how this material could be responsible for the "transforming property." Include what you know about this material and what you still need to know.

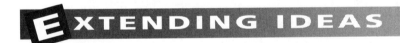

XTENDING IDEAS

▋▋N THE JOB

MEDICAL BACTERIOLOGY LABORATORY TECHNICIAN Would you be interested in using your organizational and detail-oriented skills working in the medical field? Medical bacteriology technicians conduct routine tests, which help to diagnose and treat disease, in bacteriology laboratories. A bacteriology laboratory technician can run a variety of laboratory procedures for identifying the presence of bacteria in body fluids and determining susceptibility to specific antibiotics. Technicians might prepare samples of body fluids or run laboratory tests such as urinalysis to diagnose bacterial contamination, or immune assays to detect the presence of viruses or bacteria. Technicians use light microscopes to view tissue samples and bacteria; sometimes they also use electron microscopes. This information is used by physicians, surgeons or pathologists (people who study disease) to diagnose and treat patients. Laboratory technicians usually work in a hospital or in a laboratory affiliated with a medical practice. Medical laboratory technicians might have either one or two years of post-high school education in a medical lab's training program or a two year college degree in medical lab work. A four year college degree makes it possible to become a medical technologist, who can work on specialized or more complex work and supervise a laboratory. All laboratory technicians are certified. Classes such as biology, chemistry, math, computer science, and English are necessary.

SCIENCE WRITER   With new infectious diseases and epidemics occurring around the world at an alarming rate, the job of a science writer has become closer to that of a war correspondent. Newspaper, magazine, television, and radio coverage of these events requires writers who are able to travel to other countries, report on events occurring there, translate technical scientific research and language into language that is more accessible to the general public. Good writing skills involve the readers and listeners in the drama of the moment while helping them to understand all the factors involved around crises such as epidemics. In addition to covering infectious diseases, science writers help the public keep abreast of new, exciting, and fascinating topics related to science. Besides writing for newspapers and magazines, a writer might choose to cover a topic in depth, writing about a specific discovery or spending a year in a research laboratory and writing a book about scientists, the scientific endeavor, and the topic being researched in that laboratory. Most science writers have a minimum of a college degree in a scientific discipline (although some have a liberal arts degree); they may also have a graduate level degree either in science, science journalism, or communications. Coursework in life sciences, chemistry, physics, English, and communications are recommended.

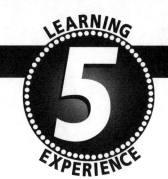

LANGUAGE OF THE CELL

PROLOGUE Imagine that you have been asked to redesign your school building. You can rearrange rooms, knock down walls, and build new wings. The first stage in the remodeling process will probably involve drawing up a plan. This plan will guide how each of the new components fits together in the new design plan and, ultimately, how the new structures will work. The plan must be clear and accurate for builders to follow.

Other sorts of plans—the play book for an athletic team, the musical score for a jazz group—work in much the same way. The information stored in the plan is read and translated into action. The information is used to construct a winning play or a resonant blend of instruments.

Avery and Griffith's work suggested that DNA might also be some sort of plan. This plan was thought to carry information that, in some way, could direct the expression of new characteristics or traits, such as a polysaccharide coat on *Diplococcus pneumoniae*. Scientists did not know what this plan looked like or how it might work.

In these situations, when the detailed workings of a biological phenomenon are a mystery, a researcher needs to start thinking creatively about the possibilities.

Figure 5.1
Musical score

What *could* it look like and how *might* it work? How do other plans work? How do they encode information? How is that information used? In this learning experience, you begin by analyzing how information is deciphered and used in two sorts of plans—a musical score that produces a particular melody, and a blueprint that produces a particular kind of house. These analogies are then applied to understanding DNA as yet another kind of plan.

Figure 5.2a
Cross section through the side of a house, with a list of construction materials

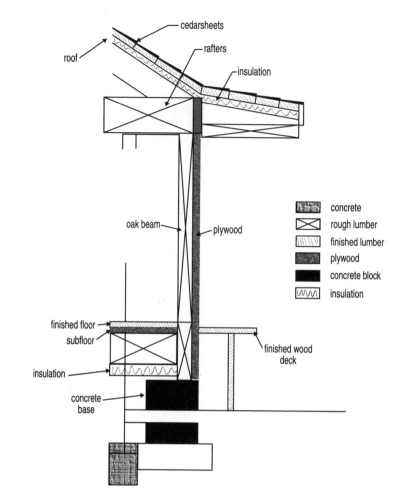

cedarsheets

roof

rafters

insulation

oak beam

plywood

concrete	
rough lumber	
finished lumber	
plywood	
concrete block	
insulation	

finished floor

subfloor

insulation

concrete base

finished wood deck

Figure 5.2b
Blueprint of house floor plan, including plans for outlets, and lighting

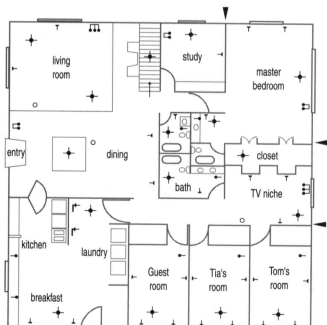

✦ Light fixture
⊥ Utility outlet
⌐ Counter height utility outlet
○ Floor outlet
▼ Flood light
← Wall switch
⊃ Two way wall switch
⊒ Three way wall switch

living room

study

master bedroom

entry

dining

closet

bath

TV niche

kitchen

laundry

breakfast

Guest room

Tia's room

Tom's room

► ANALYSIS

1. How do you go about reading music? Deciphering a floor plan? What do the plans mean? What information do you need to know to make sense of them?

2. What information do the symbols tell you about the music? the house?

3. What features remain constant within each plan? Which ones change?

4. How do the symbols relate to one another? How might the order or the placement of the symbols affect the code?

5. What features do the blueprint and the musical score have in common?

BUILDING DNA

INTRODUCTION

If DNA is responsible for conferring the characteristic of virulence on *D. pneumoniae*, can the next assumption be that DNA codes for all characteristics or traits of an organism? Does DNA itself have the characteristics necessary for such a task? How is it possible for the molecule to carry the information necessary? Researchers recognized that whatever they were looking for must have the capacity to carry an enormous amount of information—all the instructions necessary for determining the biochemical activities and specific characteristics of the cell and the organism.

Two researchers investigating the role of DNA were James Watson and Francis Crick. In 1953, they proposed a model for the structure of DNA which gave some clues as to how it might work within the cell. Their model-building process was one of trial and error, making adjustments as they learned critical pieces of evidence from other researchers. For example, Maurice Wilkins and Rosalind Franklin's work with X-ray crystallography gave important information about the spiral architecture of DNA called the "double helix."

The building blocks of DNA, termed *nucleotides*, are composed of three kinds of molecules: (1) a group of oxygen atoms clustered around a phosphorus atom (known as a *phosphate group*), (2) a simple sugar, attached to a (3) base. The base may be any one of

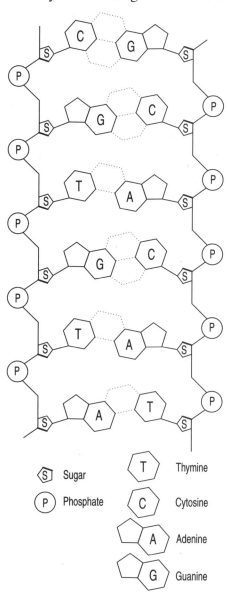

S   Sugar
P   Phosphate

T   Thymine
C   Cytosine
A   Adenine
G   Guanine

Figure 5.3
Which features remain constant in all DNA molecules? Which differ?

four rather similar nitrogen-containing bases: *adenine* (A), *thymine* (T), *guanine* (G), and *cytosine* (C).

Erwin Chargaff discovered two key "rules" which helped in figuring out how the four nucleotides were put together. Chargaff found that in the DNA of any organism examined, the number of adenine bases was always equal to the number of thymine bases, and the number of guanine bases was equal to the number of cytosine bases. This information suggested that adenine and thymine, and guanine and cytosine, might link to each other and travel in pairs. The second "rule" that Chargaff found was that the amount of adenine- and thymine-bases, as compared with cytosine- and guanine- nucleotides, varied considerably from species to species.

Many researchers at that time felt that the six molecules (the four bases and the sugar and phosphate groups) in DNA were too few to fit the task. Proteins were already known to play a central role in the vital processes of all living organisms. To many scientists, DNA could not be the hereditary "master" molecule. How could DNA carry all instructions for life with only four kinds of variable subunits?

In this activity, you will be constructing a paper model of the DNA structure Watson and Crick proposed in 1953. As you piece the molecule together, keep in mind this question: How might this molecule encode all the information necessary for determining the biochemical activities and specific characteristics of all organisms?

▶ MATERIALS NEEDED

For each group of four students:
- 1 large envelope containing copies of the following model pieces to cut out:
  - 10 of each of four bases
  - 20 phosphates
  - 20 sugars
- 4 small envelopes
- 2 paper strips (1 cm x 30 cm)
- masking tape (or drafting or other removable tape)
- white glue
- 4 scissors

▶ PROCEDURE

1. Place your group's cutouts into four separate piles—one pile for the sugar molecules, one pile for the phosphate groups, combine the adenine and thymine bases into a third pile, and combine the cytosine and guanine bases into a fourth pile. *NOTE:* Each molecule has a right and left version.

2. **STOP & THINK** Why are you combining the adenines and thymines? The cytosines and guanines?

3. Remove five bases from pile three and five bases from pile four and scramble to make a random order. Place them in a line on the left side of your lab table.

NOTE: When constructing the model, make sure the text on each molecule is facing up and can be read.

4. Remove one sugar molecule from the sugar pile to attach to one of the bases. Glue the tab on the sugar (as a bond) to the lower corner of the base. (Look for the letter S at the corner of the base.) (See Figure 5.4.)

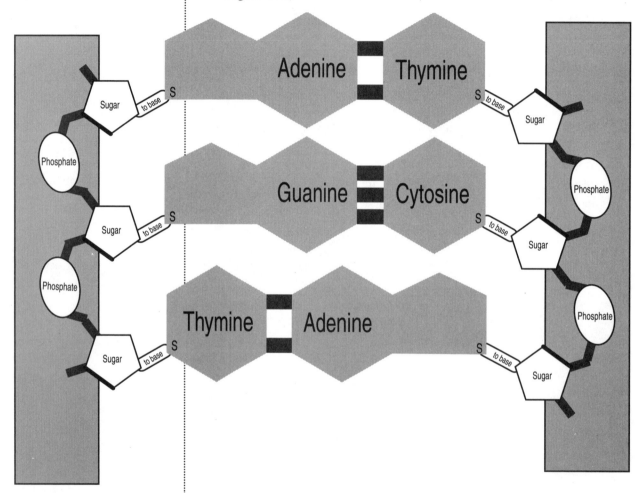

Figure 5.4
DNA model constructed with paper sides.

5. Remove one phosphate group from its pile to attach to the bonded sugar molecule. Glue the tabs.

6. Locate the appropriate matching (complementary) base from pile three or four to attach to the model. Attach the two bases by taping the "hydrogen bond" tabs together. (There are two bonds between Adenine and Thymine, and three bonds between Cytosine and Guanine).

7. 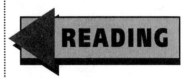 Read the Analysis questions that follow this procedure and discuss them with your group as you construct your model.

8. Repeat steps 3–6 for each of the bases lined up on the left side of your table, making ten complete sets of base pairs.

9. Complete the model by gluing the model to the two paper strips (see Figure 5.4).

▶ ANALYSIS

As you and your group construct the model, discuss your responses to the following questions:

1. Describe the basic features of a DNA molecule. What information do the letter symbols give you?

2. What features of the DNA molecule remain constant in various organisms? What features differ?

3. How do the nucleotides connect to one another? How might the order or the placement of bases affect the code?

Write responses to the following questions in your notebook:

4. Write the sequence of bases for the DNA strand you constructed.

5. If 27% of the bases in a certain segment of DNA were adenine, what would be the percentages of thymine, cytosine, and guanine?

6. If DNA determines the characteristics of pneumococci, it seems possible that DNA could determine the traits of all living things. This means that DNA must be able to carry an enormous amount of information. How can a molecule composed of only four different kinds of subunits carry large amounts of diverse information?

7. How might DNA differ among different organisms; for example, how do you think mouse DNA or bacterial DNA differ from human DNA?

WRITING THE BOOK OF LIFE

READING

When Watson and Crick announced their model of the double helix in 1953, they described an extraordinary instruction "book" packed inside the nuclei of all our cells. Written in a language of few letters (four nucleotides), DNA contains all the information needed for the maintenance and perpetuation of life.

What roles were played by each of the component pieces—the sugars, the phosphates, and the bases—was the critical question Watson and Crick faced as they created and revised their DNA model. They knew they needed a pattern that could be written in thousands of variations. Yet a choice of only three pieces (sugar, phosphate, and base) did not initially seem to provide many options.

In the following excerpt, Crick (1954) describes his analysis of this elegant molecule:

Excerpted from

The Structure of the Hereditary Material

F.H.C. Crick, Scientific American, October 1954, pages 54–61.

...It is now known that DNA consists of a very long chain made up of alternate sugar and phosphate groups. The sugar is always the same sugar, known as deoxyribose. And it is always joined onto the phosphate in the same way, so that the long chain is perfectly regular, repeating the same phosphate-sugar sequence over and over again.

But while the phosphate-sugar chain is perfectly regular, the molecule as a whole is not, because each sugar has a "base" attached to it and the base is not always the same. Four different types of bases are commonly found: ...adenine and guanine... thymine and cytosine... So far as is known the order in which they follow one another along the chain is irregular, and probably varies from one piece of DNA to another. In fact, we suspect that the order of the bases is what confers specificity on a given DNA.

...we found that we could not arrange the bases any way we pleased; the four bases would fit into the structure only in certain pairs. In any pair, there must be one big one [the *purines*

adenine and guanine] and one little one [the *pyrimidines* thymine and cytosine]. A pair of pyrimidines is too short to bridge the gap between the two chains, and a pair of purines is too big to fit into the space.

Adenine must always be paired with thymine, and guanine with cytosine; it is impossible to fit the bases together in any other combination in our model.... The model places no restriction, however, on the sequence of pairs along the structure. Any specified pair can follow any other. This is because a pair of bases is flat, and since in this model they are stacked roughly like a pile of coins, it does not matter which pair goes above which....

...the exciting thing about a model of this type is that it immediately suggests how the DNA might produce an exact copy of itself. The model consists of two parts, each of which is the complement of the other. Thus either chain may act as a sort of mold on which a complementary chain can be synthesized. The two chains of a DNA, let us say, unwind and separate. Each begins to build a new complement onto itself. When the process is completed, there are two pairs of chains where we had only one. Moreover, because of the specific pairing of the bases the sequence of the pairs of bases will have been duplicated exactly; in other words, the mold has not only assembled the building blocks but has put them together in just the right order.

Let us imagine that we have a single helical chain of DNA, and that floating around it inside the cell is a supply of precursors of the four sorts of building blocks needed to make a new chain...from time to time, a loose unit will attach itself by its base to one of the bases of the single DNA chain. Another loose unit may attach itself to an adjoining base on the chain. Now if one or both of the two newly attached units is not the correct mate for the one it has joined on the chain, the two newcomers will be unable to link together, because they are not the right

distance apart. One or both will soon drift away, to be replaced by other units. When, however, two adjacent newcomers are the correct partners for their opposite numbers on the chain, they will be in just the right position to be linked together and begin to form a new chain. Thus only the unit with the proper base will gain a permanent hold at any given position, and eventually the right partners will fill in the vacancies all along the forming chain. While this is going on, the other single chain of the original pair also will be forming a new chain complementary to itself.

...We suspect that the sequence of the bases acts as a kind of genetic code. Such an arrangement can carry an enormous amount of information. If we imagine that the pairs of bases correspond to the dots and dashes of the Morse code, there is enough DNA in a single cell of the human body to encode about 1,000 large textbooks...

The following figures illustrate several important ideas about the structure of DNA that Crick suggested in his article.

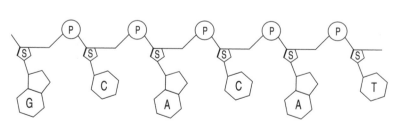

Figure 5.5
Crick's description of the DNA chain sounded much like a long chain made of links. This chain was formed by the sugar-phosphate backbone. From each of these links, bases were suspended. Each link with its base constituted a nucleotide subunit.

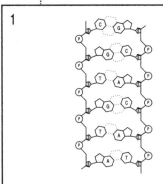

Cytosine

Guanine

Figure 5.6
The relationship between the purines (adenine and guanine) and the pyrimidines (thymine and cytosine). Adenine always pairs with thymine; guanine always pairs with cytosine.

Adenine

Thymine

Figure 5.7
The model proposed by Watson and Crick suggests how DNA might produce an exact copy of itself.

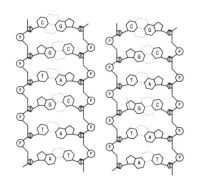

1	2
DNA consists of two chains.	DNA chains unwind and separate.
3	4
Each chain builds a new complement of itself by pairing bases.	When process is complete, there are two pairs of chains exactly alike.

Although Watson and Crick's model provided a giant leap in our understanding, a big question remained: How can a set of characters embedded in DNA actually determine what our bodies do? What could something like AGTCAT mean?

DNA as a Coded Plan

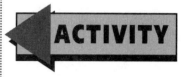

INTRODUCTION   You began this learning experience with the questions: For what functions does your DNA plan? How might a DNA plan work?

When Watson and Crick published their model, they suggested that the sequence of the bases in DNA might act as a code. Although they were not sure at that time what DNA coded for, they thought it was intriguing that the structures of DNA and proteins were based on the same general plan. This plan included a regular, repeating backbone. The plan's variation came from the sequence of the bases of the nucleotides or the sidegroups of the amino acids.

With this new knowledge, protein and DNA researchers thought back to Griffith's transformation experiment. The protein researchers had argued that making a polysaccharide coat required enzymes to put the right building blocks together in the right arrangement. They believed that nothing in the cell could be built without the enzymes directing and facilitating the construction work. If a polysaccharide coat were built, proteins must be involved. The DNA researchers stood behind Avery's evidence that DNA was the transforming material.

When DNA and proteins were found to have such similar chemical arrangements, these two fields of research came together. Watson and Crick suggested that the four bases of the DNA might code for the 20 amino acids that make up the proteins of cells. In this light, the change in characteristics of the pneumococci did require the *work* of proteins. But it was the *plan* of the DNA that determined the protein would be made. The plan carried the information that directed which protein would be produced. That protein set to work to make the polysaccharide coat.

How exactly could this happen? How do the symbols of DNA contain the information for proteins? Crick suggested that the base symbols of DNA could be analogous to the dots and dashes of the Morse code. The Morse code uses only two symbols to represent all 26 letters, ten numbers, and a few punctuation marks. Placed in combinations of one to six symbols long for each letter or number, a set of symbols can make words and phrases. In turn, an infinite number of messages can be created.

A	• —	N	— •	1	• — — — —
B	— • • •	O	— — —	2	• • — — —
C	— • — •	P	• — — •	3	• • • — —
D	— • •	Q	— — • —	4	• • • • —
E	•	R	• — •	5	• • • • •
F	• • — •	S	• • •	6	— • • • •
G	— — •	T	—	7	— — • • •
H	• • • •	U	• • —	8	— — — • •
I	• •	V	• • • —	9	— — — — •
J	• — — —	W	• — —	0	— — — — —
K	— • —	X	— • • —	.	• — • — • —
L	• — • •	Y	— • — —	,	— — • • — —
M	— —	Z	— — • •	?	• • — — • •

► TASK

Write responses to the following in your notebook:

1. Try writing your name in code, using the symbol system Morse set up.

2. Working in pairs, write a short sentence to your partner. When you are finished, swap sentences and try to decode your partner's message.

3. What similarities are there between Morse code and DNA? How might this apply to the way DNA and proteins work? In a short essay, explain what you know so far about the molecular languages of DNA and proteins. The following questions might help you to get started:

   a. Describe the makeup of these languages.

   b. How does one "speak" and make sense in each of these languages?

   c. How might the DNA alphabet be translated into the protein alphabet?

   d. How might DNA determine what a cell does?

4. Construct a concept map for DNA. Include the following terms: transforming factor, information, nucleotides, sugar, phosphate group, base pairs, building blocks, adenine, thymine, guanine, cytosine. Use additional terms as you need them.

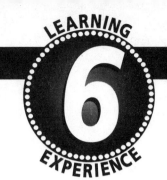

NUCLEIC ACID TO PROTEIN

PROLOGUE **D**NA stores the information of the cell; proteins are the biomolecules that make the cell. What is the relationship between these two biomolecules?

Stored information is just that: information that is in storage, waiting to be used. Information in the blueprints for a house awaits the construction team that can translate the symbols and diagrams into the substance of a house; the notes in musical scores only come to life when the musician translates the notes into the complexity of musical sounds. How is the information in DNA, specifically in the sequence of its nucleotides, translated into proteins which, in turn, carry out many functions?

In this learning experience, you will be exploring the cellular processes in which the information in DNA is expressed as the protein the cell needs to carry out all of its functions.

THE MESSENGER TELLS ALL

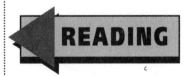

If DNA is found in the nucleus and protein is made in the cytoplasm (as we now know it is), a logistical problem seems to exist. In 1957, shortly after describing the double helical structure of DNA, Francis Crick hypothesized that there needed to exist an intermediate translator of the information between DNA and protein, something that could carry the information from the DNA in the nucleus to the site of protein synthesis in the cytoplasm. The "central dogma", as it came to be known, stated that information stored in DNA was carried by another kind of molecule. In 1960 this "other molecule" was identified as another kind of nucleic acid, *ribonucleic acid* or

RNA (see Figure 6.1). In ensuing years, scientists learned that, in general, only one strand of the DNA double helix was copied into RNA.

Figure 6.1
The information in DNA is used to assemble proteins.

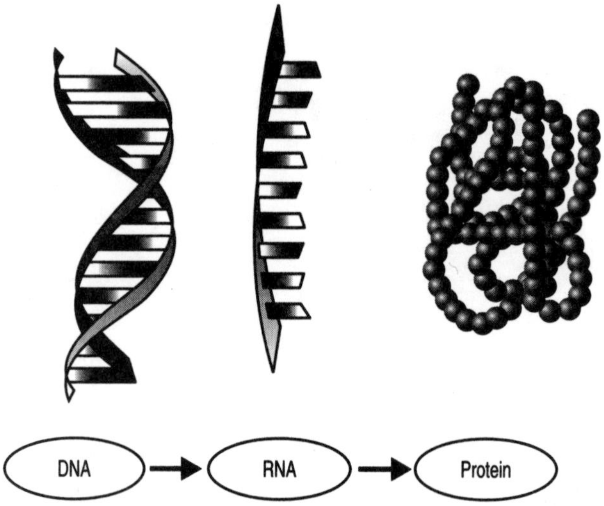

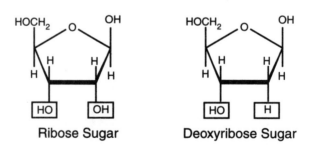

The role of RNA is essential. Just as monks copied or "transcribed" writings of manuscripts for distribution in medieval times, the information in DNA is transcribed or copied into RNA molecules which look very similar to the original but have several characteristics which distinguish RNA from DNA.

RNA almost always consists of a single strand, not a double helix. Another significant difference between RNA and DNA is the sugar. RNA contains the sugar ribose instead of the deoxyribose sugar found in DNA. The structures in Figure 6.2 indicate the difference in the sugar component of the two types of nucleic acids.

Figure 6.2
RNA is chemically like DNA except for its sugars. Each ribose has an additional oxygen atom compared with deoxyribose. Note the presence and the location of the oxygen in the sugar of the RNA and DNA molecules.

A further difference between RNA and DNA is in the composition of one of their bases: DNA has thymine; instead of thymine RNA has the base *uracil*. The difference in these bases is shown in Figure 6.3.

Transcription is the process by which information encoded in DNA is transferred to an RNA molecule. The information must be copied because DNA does not leave the nucleus. Just as an architect might protect building blueprints from loss or damage by keeping them in a safe or locked place, your cells protect DNA by keeping it safe in

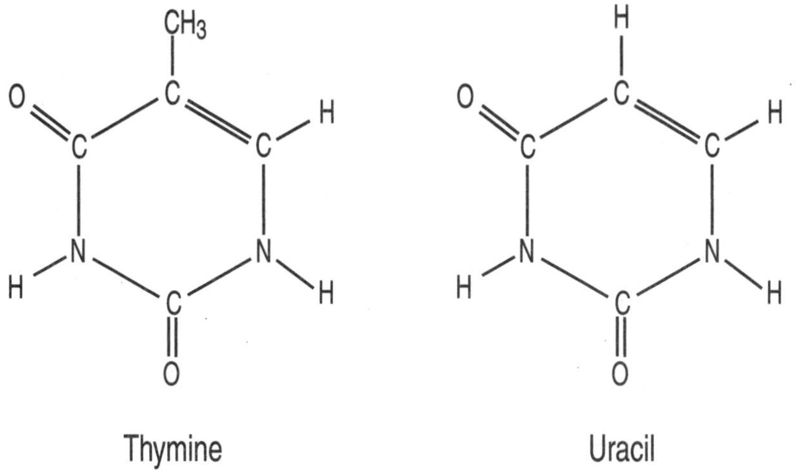

Thymine   Uracil

Figure 6.3
The difference between thymine and uracil

the nucleus. Instead, copies of the DNA are made and then sent into the cell's cytoplasm. These copies are the RNA. The RNA then directs the assembly of proteins.

The process of transcription is similar to replication. The DNA chains unwind and separate. The chain begins to build a complement of itself using RNA nucleotides present in the nucleus. Each DNA base is paired with its complementary RNA base. Cytosine is paired with guanine, but because RNA contains uracil instead of thymine, adenine is paired with uracil. In this way, the RNA strand is gradually built. In general, only one of the DNA strands has information to be used for the protein and, therefore, only this strand is copied into RNA. This DNA strand is called the *"sense" strand*. (As you might guess, the other strand is called the *"anti-sense" strand*.)

After transcription of the DNA is complete, the newly transcribed RNA leaves the nucleus. It passes through pores or openings in the nuclear membrane into the cytoplasm, where it then begins to direct the assembly of proteins. This molecule is called *messenger RNA (mRNA)*. RNA also plays other roles in the cell, as you will see. Its chemical characteristics and structure enable it to move readily from the nucleus to the cytoplasm. RNA is also more easily broken down (degraded) than DNA. This feature gives the cell a great deal of flexibility and control in what information it expresses as protein. When the cell no longer has need of the information encoded in a particular sequence of DNA, it can stop transcribing it into RNA by various control mechanisms. The RNA already in the cell will eventually be degraded and the cell will no longer make that protein and, therefore, will not express that characteristic.

▶ ANALYSIS

1. Why is it that the information encoded in the DNA is transcribed into RNA and then translated rather than being translated directly?

2. Describe how each of the building blocks for DNA (see Figure 6.4) differs from those for RNA.

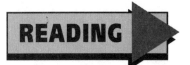

Phosphate Group

Base

P

B

S

Sugar

Figure 6.4
DNA nucleotide

3. Envision an organism that had no DNA, that used RNA only. How might such a system carry out the transfer of information? What might be the advantages of such a system? The disadvantages?

4. Use the DNA model you created in Learning Experience 5. Separate the strands of the model by separating the chains along the central hydrogen bonds. Choose one strand of DNA as the sense strand and determine the sequence of its mRNA.

READING

CRACKING THE GENETIC CODE

In 1961, Marshall Nirenberg figured out how information was stored in DNA. He "cracked the code" by introducing an mRNA strand consisting solely of uracil nucleotides (as in UUUUUUUUU) into an extract of broken cells which was capable of making proteins in a test tube. From this sequence he obtained a protein made entirely of a single kind of amino acid, phenylalanine. When an mRNA containing the sequence AAAAAAAAA was placed in the tube, a protein consisting of another single amino acid type, lysine, was obtained. All possible RNA sequence combinations were tried. Using this approach, scientists were able to determine that the nucleic acid code in DNA occurred in triplets; that is, a series of three nucleotides in RNA (such as UGA) specifies a particular amino acid. Each nucleotide triplet is called a *codon*.

Using Nirenberg's technique, scientists were able to decipher the code for all 20 amino acids. The result of all this work is the decoder of protein synthesis, the codon table in Table 6.5. With the aid of this table, the amino acids encoded in the RNA can be identified. The sequence of the bases in each codon determines which amino acid will be added next to a growing protein chain. In turn, the sequence of amino acids will determine the shape and, ultimately, the function of that protein.

▶ **ANALYSIS**

1. Use Table 6.5 to decode the triplet AUG. Try decoding a few more by jotting down any triplet of RNA nucleotides and seeing if you can decode it. Does it seem as if all triplets have a corresponding amino acid? How do you know?

	G = guanine
	C = cytosine
	A = adenine
	U = uracil

codons	GCA GCC GCG GCU	AGA AGG CGA CGC CGG CGU	AAC AAU	GAC GAU	UGC UGU	CAA CAG	GAA GAG
Abbreviations for amino acids	ala	arg	asn	asp	cys	gln	glu

codons	GGA GGC GGG GGU	CAC CAU	AUA AUC AUU	UUA UUG CUA CUC CUG CUU	AAA AAG	AUG	UUC UUU	CCA CCC CCG CCU
Abbreviations for amino acids	gly	his	ile	leu	lys	met	phe	pro

codons	AGC AGU UCA UCC UCG UCU	ACA ACC ACG ACU	UGG	UAC UAU	GUA GUC GUG GUU	UAA UAG UGA
Abbreviations for amino acids	ser	thr	trp	tyr	val	stop

Table 6.5
Each amino acid is coded for by three mRNA bases arranged in a specific sequence called a codon.

For ease of writing, the 20 amino acids can be abbreviated as follows:

ala	alanine	gly	glycine	pro	proline
arg	arginine	his	histidine	ser	serine
asn	asparagine	ile	isoleucine	thr	threonine
asp	aspartic acid	leu	leucine	trp	tryptophan
cys	cysteine	lys	lysine	tyr	tyrosine
gln	glutamine	met	methionine	val	valine
glu	glutamic acid	phe	phenylalanine		

2. All communication needs punctuation. Which codons represent punctuation?

3. Find the amino acids encoded by UCU, UCC, and UCA. What do you observe? What does this mean?

DANCES WITH RIBOSOMES

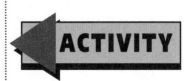

INTRODUCTION   If DNA is the master blueprint of the cell, and RNA molecules are the copies to be distributed as the guide to the building process, then the components of the protein synthesis machinery are the construction team. The *ribosome* is the site of protein synthesis and is the structure that holds all the pieces in place. Found in the cytoplasm, the ribosome is comprised of about 50 different kinds of proteins all wrapped up in a structural RNA. The ribosome has a special place where mRNAs bind.

Transfer RNAs (tRNA) are the actual translators of the code. These are a group of RNAs that have a twisted loop structure made up of nucleotides. At the loop end there are three nucleotides (*anticodons*) which match the sequence of a codon triplet in the mRNA; at the other end is an amino acid, bound to the tRNA. Figure 6.6 shows an example of tRNA. The codon sequence in the mRNA would be UUU. The anticodon on the tRNA is therefore AAA and the amino acid at the other end would be phenylalanine. The sequence at the end of the tRNA loop matches the mRNA sequence (much the way two strands of the DNA sequence match) and brings along with it its amino acid.

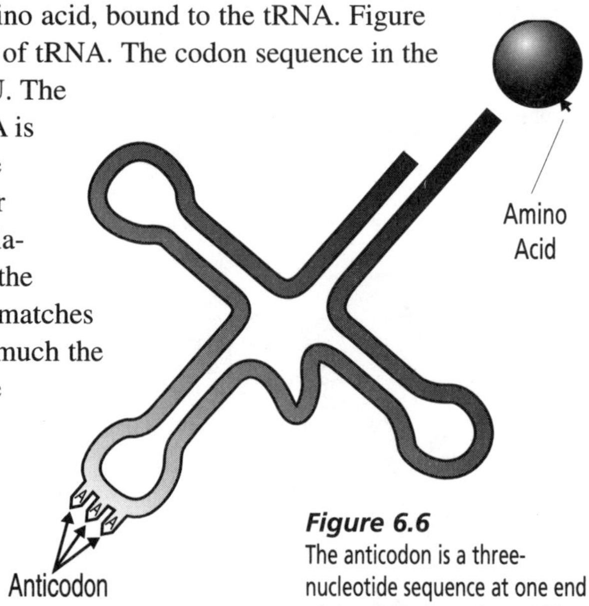

Amino Acid

Anticodon

Figure 6.6
The anticodon is a three-nucleotide sequence at one end of the tRNA. An amino acid is attached at the opposite end.

In this activity, you will model protein synthesis. You and your classmates will take on the various roles of the protein synthesis machinery. The classroom represents the cytoplasm, and the corridor outside the classroom represents the nucleus.

▶ ROLES

- mRNA:
  2–3 students become the
  single strand of mRNA

- ribosome: 1 student is the ribosome

- enzymes which assemble amino acids into a protein chain: 2 students with tape and string

- transfer RNA (4 different types, multiple copies of each—GAC, CUU, AAA, and UUC—each of which holds an inflated balloon (amino acid) to which it is color coded): remaining students in the class.

The Procedure describes, in detail, the process of protein synthesis. Once you have assumed your role, you and your classmates will create a protein as a class. It is important that you understand each step in the process. This "central dogma" of biology is essential to all living things. The information stored in DNA flows through RNA to protein and these proteins are essential for carrying out the functions and determining the characteristics of an organism. In the case of the bacteria *Diplococcus pneumoniae*, the DNA transferred from the virulent bacteria caused the nonvirulent bacteria to make a protein which made it pathogenic to the host.

▶ PROCEDURE

1. The mRNA starts in the corridor (nucleus) and enters the cytoplasm (classroom).

2. The mRNA attaches to the ribosome which has been structured to reveal three nucleotide symbols (a codon) at a time. As mRNA moves through the ribosome, the person holding the ribosome calls out the revealed codon.

3. The appropriate tRNA with the complementary anticodon comes up to the ribosome bringing its attached amino acid (balloon).

4. The enzymes take the balloon from the tRNA and tape it to the string that they are holding.

5. The mRNA continues to move through the ribosome exposing each codon.

6. Appropriate tRNAs bring balloons (amino acids) that continue to be added to the protein chain. When tRNA gives up its amino acid balloon, it goes to pick up the appropriate free amino acids until it will again be needed. Free amino acids (uninflated balloons) will be stored in a designated area in the room (cytoplasm) where they may be retrieved by a tRNA that has released its amino acid (balloon) to the growing protein chain on the ribosome.

7. When the complete chain of amino acids has been assembled, the enzymes will detach the chain from the ribosome and suspend it where it will be visible to the entire class.

▶ ANALYSIS

1. Create a concept map that summarizes protein synthesis—the process by which information is transferred from DNA to protein in the cell. Use the following terms in your map: nucleus, cytoplasm, ribosome, transcription, translation, DNA, mRNA, tRNA, amino acid, protein,

enzyme. Be sure to include other terms from this module.

2. Suppose the mRNA "message" that leaves the nucleus and attaches to the ribosome were changed so that the final codon was GUA instead of the existing GAA. What would be the composition of the resulting protein chain?

3. What would be the nucleotide composition of the DNA sense strand that produced the change in mRNA?

4. What would be the nucleotide composition of the DNA sense strand that produced the original mRNA?

5. Using your answers to questions 2, 3, and 4, determine how the original double-stranded DNA molecule could have changed to produce the new messenger RNA. Such a change in DNA is called a *mutation*. You are being asked to figure out specifically what mutation in DNA might have occurred to produce the changes in RNA and the protein chain that is ultimately produced.

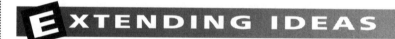

EXTENDING IDEAS

ON THE JOB

GENETICIST   Are you interested in how traits are passed from one generation to another? Geneticists are scientists who study how biological traits originate and how they are passed from one generation to the next in various life forms. Geneticists usually specialize by studying one particular type of organism such as plants, animals or other organisms. Plant geneticists plant seeds and then grow the plants to maturity in order to look at both chromosome structure and chromosome number of a cell, to use equipment to identify the gene sequence of a particular piece of DNA, or to look for variations from one species to another. Once the location of genes has been identified on the chromosomes, geneticists might insert the gene into a cell and in tissue culture replicate the gene sequence so there are many copies of it. Molecular biologists or genetic engineers are able to manipulate the gene sequence. Geneticists studying animal organisms also watch the animals grow to maturity and then look at both chromosome structure and number of a cell to either identify the locations of specific genes or to look for variations from one species to another. The laboratory techniques and procedures used by molecular biologists are not unique to molecular biology, but are the techniques and tools used by chemists and cell biologists. For someone with a high school degree or a two year college degree, positions as a laboratory technician are available. A four year college degree makes it possible to be a laboratory assistant or research geneticist. With a master's or doctoral degree, geneticists can teach in a university or pursue independent research in a university or laboratory. Classes such as biology, chemistry, math, English, and computer science are necessary.

TEACHER   Do you like sharing what you know about microorganisms or how disease is caused? Teachers combine their knowledge of a subject with the ability to make it interesting and communicate clearly. Teachers at all grade levels would plan what topics to cover and what activities or labs to use to illustrate the topic, prepare activities or labs (this includes collecting all the materials and setting up the activity), work with students as they do the activities, write and grade quizzes and tests. A teacher who works in an elementary school might teach one class all subjects, including science, or could just teach science and work with all the classes in the school. Elementary school science consists of lots of activities and encouraging students to ask a lot of questions and wonder about the world. A middle school science teacher teaches general science courses which focus on science as a way of thinking and continues to build on the concepts students explored in elementary school. High school science teachers most often teach in one particular subject area (biology, chemistry or physics), although many are versatile and can teach in several subject areas. High school science explores science concepts in depth and also looks at the science within social, historical, ethical, and political contexts. Not all science teachers work in a school. Some work in museums, zoos, aquariums or science centers, teaching the general public and taking classes on school field trips. A minimum of a four year college degree is required with classes in your subject area and the completion of a teacher preparation program. The teacher preparation program includes courses on child development and on teaching methods as well as student teaching. Requirements for teacher certification vary from state to state. Some teachers have a master's degree in education or science education. Classes in subjects such as biology, chemistry, physics, mathematics, English, and psychology are recommended.

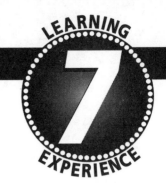

PROTEIN, THE WONDER INGREDIENT

PROLOGUE The experiments of Griffith and of Avery and his colleagues demonstrated that DNA contained information enabling the bacteria *Diplococcus pneumoniae* to produce a polysaccharide capsule, and that this capsule allowed the bacteria to grow and flourish in the host, which would exhibit the symptoms of pneumonia.

What is the relationship between DNA and the ability of *D. pneumoniae* to synthesize a protective capsule? In the last learning experience, you explored the processes involved in the translation of information from DNA into protein. The difference between the nonvirulent and virulent strains was actually a difference in just one enzyme—the virulent strain contained a specific enzyme that enabled it to synthesize a polysaccharide capsule. The information that was transferred, transforming a nonvirulent strain to a virulent strain, was in the DNA code. Because it enabled the non-virulent strain to produce the enzyme that could then facilitate the synthesis of the polysaccharide capsule, the presence of this DNA sequence determined that this strain would now be virulent (see Figure 7.1).

Figure 7.1
Transforming factor makes a new enzyme.

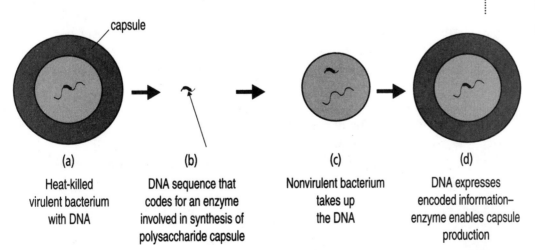

capsule

(a)	(b)	(c)	(d)
Heat-killed virulent bacterium with DNA	DNA sequence that codes for an enzyme involved in synthesis of polysaccharide capsule	Nonvirulent bacterium takes up the DNA	DNA expresses encoded information–enzyme enables capsule production

Proteins are essential components of all living organisms and can carry out enormously diverse functions. How do proteins do what they do? What makes them uniquely able to carry out a wide range of functions, thereby directing a great variety of chemical activities? In this learning experience, you will explore the function of these wondrous molecules and examine how their structure permits them to carry out these functions.

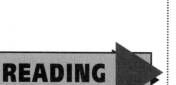

PROTEIN, PROTEIN, EVERYWHERE

Living organisms contain an immense assortment of biomolecules. The simplest life forms, bacteria, contain about 5,000 different biomolecules, including 3,000 different kinds of proteins. In humans, the numbers and the variation are even greater. It is this diversity of protein biomolecules that enables cells to carry out the myriad of activities involved in life processes. Proteins are a good example of the simplicity within diversity; they are all chains of amino acids. It is the number and order of the amino acid subunits that result in the diversity of proteins; this diversity then determines differences in characteristics of cells, and therefore of whole organisms.

Each type of protein is superbly efficient at one task. How many proteins exist in the human body? No one knows, but a hundred thousand is not a bad guess, and though none of these protein molecules is identical to any found in bacteria, some of their functions are quite similar.

What are these proteins? Why are there so many different kinds? What do they do and how do they do it? Actually, you are probably familiar with proteins—they are the "wonder ingredients" in products you use every day, such as the laundry detergents that claim they can get out your toughest stains, and shampoos that are supposed to make your hair look terrific.

You may be most familiar with the proteins in the foods you eat. Proteins are an essential part of your daily diet. Plants can make their proteins from carbon dioxide, water, nitrates, sulfates, and phosphates; animals, on the other hand, can synthesize only a limited number of proteins and are mainly dependent on plants or other animals as dietary sources of protein. Protein intake is required regularly in animals because their bodies have little stored protein. If excess protein is taken in, more than the body can use, it is stored as fat.

Proteins are essential to the structure and function of all living organisms. Next to water, protein is the most abundant substance in cells. Proteins make up half of the solid matter in cells (water makes up 70% of the cell) and perform a wide variety of tasks in organisms. These tasks can be classified by biological function.

The largest class of proteins consists of the *enzymes*, protein mole-

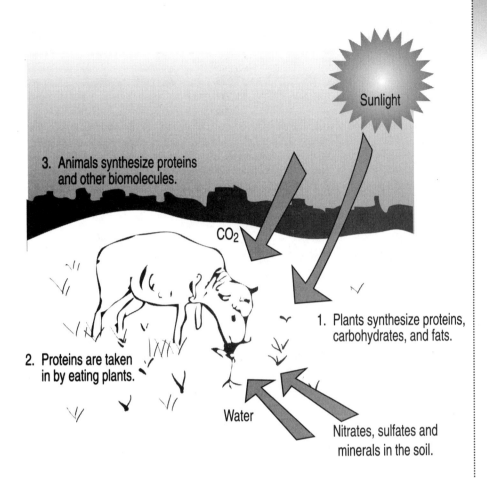

3. Animals synthesize proteins and other biomolecules.

Sunlight

CO_2

2. Proteins are taken in by eating plants.

1. Plants synthesize proteins, carbohydrates, and fats.

Water

Nitrates, sulfates and minerals in the soil.

Figure 7.2
Protein flow in nature

cules that facilitate and enhance the rate of chemical reactions in the cell. That is, enzymes assist in chemical reactions so that the reactions proceed with speed and efficiency. Without enzymes, the metabolic reactions of the cell would still take place but far too slowly to sustain life; it would take you about 50 years to digest your lunch. Reactions such as those involved in the breakdown of food, the synthesis of cell components, or the transport and storage of energy that otherwise might take days or weeks or years to happen, occur in milliseconds in the cell because of the action of enzymes. Examples of enzymes include: lactase which breaks down the milk sugar lactose into glucose and galactose; catalase which degrades hydrogen peroxide to oxygen and water; RNA polymerase which is responsible for transcribing the information in DNA into mRNA; and diphosphoribulose carboxylase which fixes carbon dioxide (CO_2) into sugar in photosynthetic organisms. Note that the suffix -ase is usually found in an enzyme's name.

The second major class of proteins makes up the structural components of cells and tissues. Collagen, the major structural protein in connective tissue and in bone, is also part of the "glue" that binds a group of cells together to form a tissue. Another structural protein, keratin, gives strength to skin, hair, nails, horns, and feathers.

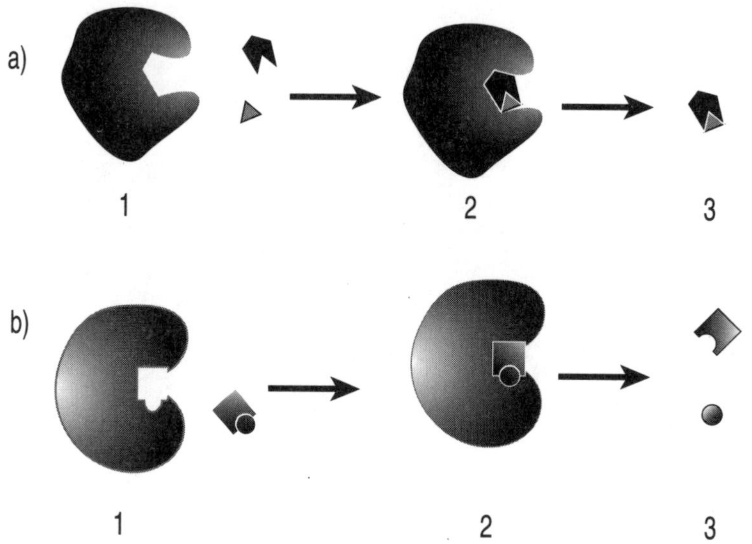

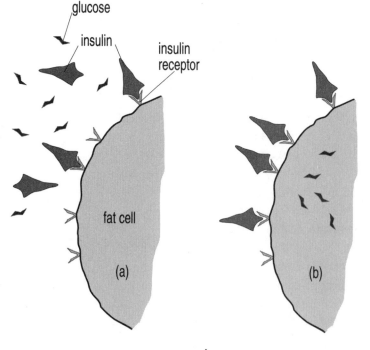

Figure 7.3
Enzymes facilitate anabolism (a) by putting molecules together and (b) facilitate catabolism by taking molecules apart.

Figure 7.4
(a) Insulin binds to a protein receptor on fat cells (b) causing the cells to take up glucose from the blood.

glucose

insulin

insulin receptor

fat cell

(a)

(b)

In addition, proteins carry out other essential types of functions. Actin and myosin are the two major proteins that enable muscles to contract. Some proteins have a transport function: hemoglobin in blood carries oxygen around the body; myoglobin transports oxygen through muscle tissue; and serum albumin transports fatty acids through the blood to various organs. Hormones such as insulin (which regulates blood sugar) and somatotropin (a growth hormone) are proteins. Proteins found in the immune system, such as antibodies, protect us from infection. In contrast, toxins—proteins made by organisms including bacteria, plants, and snakes—may do us great harm.

Many proteins act by binding to other proteins and triggering a specific cellular response. For example, the hormone insulin controls the level of glucose in the blood. Insulin acts by binding to specific proteins on the surface of muscle, liver, and fat cells. This binding causes a change in their cell membranes that results in their taking up glucose from the blood, thus reducing the concentration of blood glucose (see Figure 7.4).

Proteins also can serve as a source of energy for cells. If the diet does not supply enough fat and carbohydrate, which are the primary sources of energy in the cell, stored fat is broken down for energy. But if stored fat is used up, as in starvation or extreme dieting,

Learning Experience 7   Protein, the Wonder Ingredient

then proteins can be used for energy, instead, even at the expense of building new cells and maintaining tissue structure.

How do proteins carry out all of these essential functions? How does the structure of a protein relate to its function? The shape of an individual protein is very important in its function. All proteins have a linear sequence of amino acids, but the molecules are folded into complex three-dimensional structures. The shapes of these structures are determined by which amino acids make up the proteins and the sequence in which they occur. Just looking at the sequence of amino acids in a protein cannot tell us how it folds; it cannot tell us how growth hormone makes us taller or how a bacterial toxin can kill us. But the information in that sequence plays an essential role in determining if and how these interactions take place. Exactly how the sequence of amino acids determines a protein's function is not completely understood, but some of the pieces of the puzzle have been determined, as you will see in your investigation.

LIVER AND LET LIVER

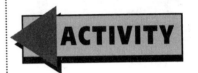

INTRODUCTION   Liver may not be one of your favorite foods, but the liver in your own body should be one of your favorite organs. It plays the life-saving function of detoxification. Every day your body takes in toxic substances from the air and the food you eat. In addition, some of the byproducts of your cells' metabolic activities are toxic to your system. The job of the liver is to neutralize and dispose of these toxic substances—a sort of hazardous waste disposal. Without a liver, hazardous products would soon build up, inhibit vital metabolic processes, and result in death.

One of these toxic metabolic byproducts in animal tissues is a molecule called hydrogen peroxide. You may be familiar with hydrogen peroxide as a substance which can be used for bleaching hair or for disinfecting wounds to prevent infection. Hydrogen peroxide (H_2O_2) is toxic to living things because it produces something called a superoxide radical, O_2^-, from oxygen. This radical can destroy certain biomolecules such as proteins. Therefore, it is essential that organisms be able to dispose of hydrogen peroxide. Catalase is an enzyme present in liver cells (and other plant and animal cells) that neutralizes this hazardous waste product by breaking it down into harmless molecules. In the following investigation, you will examine the activity of catalase.

▶ MATERIALS NEEDED

For each pair of students:

- 2 pairs of safety goggles
- 2 small pieces of liver (one cooked and one raw)
- 2 flasks (125- to 250-mL) or test tubes (13 x 100 mm)
- 2 balloons
- 50–100 mL hydrogen peroxide

▶ PROCEDURE

1. Place raw liver in one flask or test tube and cooked liver in another flask.

2. Pour enough hydrogen peroxide into each flask to cover each piece of liver.

3. If possible, cover the top of each flask or test tube with a balloon to capture the gas which is being formed.

4. Observe the reaction for 5–10 minutes. Write your observations in your notebook and write responses to the following Analysis questions.

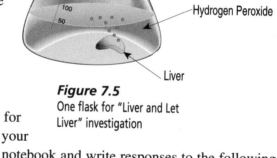

Figure 7.5
One flask for "Liver and Let Liver" investigation

▶ ANALYSIS

1. What happened when hydrogen peroxide was added to the raw liver?

2. The chemical formula for hydrogen peroxide is H_2O_2. What gas do you think was produced? How might you identify the gas?

3. What else might have been produced?

4. Write a chemical equation which describes what happened.

5. How was the reaction in the cooked liver different from the reaction in the raw liver?

6. Based on your knowledge from the readings, what was the cause of the difference in these two reactions?

Learning Experience 7   Protein, the Wonder Ingredient

GETTING INTO SHAPE

INTRODUCTION   The first step in most protein reactions is for one protein to bind to another molecule. In the case of enzymes, this binding step brings the second molecule, which could be another protein, a sugar, a lipid, or a nucleic acid, into position so that the enzyme can act on it. Transport proteins, such as hemoglobin and certain membrane proteins, bind molecules in order to move them from place to place. Structural proteins, such as collagen, may bind to one another to give shape and strength to the structure.

These binding interactions occur at specific sites on the protein molecules (*binding sites*). The binding site on a protein is defined by the shape of the protein. The folding of the protein results in a groove, cleft, or pocket on its surface into which the second molecule fits, much like a key in a lock. If the shape of this binding site is altered, the ability of the protein to interact with the second molecule may be lost, rendering the protein unable to carry out its function. Once the second molecule binds to the protein, that enzyme can then do its job, whether that is an enzymatic reaction, a transport function, a structural function, or something else.

The principles of *protein folding* are one of the important, unsolved mysteries of science. It is known so far that the amino acid composition and the order in which these amino acids occur in the protein play a central role in determining how a protein will fold. Amino acids have a characteristic structure and differ from one another in their side groups, which may have a positive, negative, or neutral charge (see Figure 7.6). The positive and negative charges on the amino acids appear to be important in folding. Amino acids also demonstrate *hydrophobic* (water-fearing) and *hydrophilic* (water-loving) properties seen in lipids. These properties are also important in folding, as the water-fearing parts tend to move to the interior of the molecule, away from the water. Another factor involved in folding is the ability of amino acids to form chemical bridges or bonds between each other.

In this activity, you will build a model that demonstrates the first step in protein function, the binding of a protein to another molecule.

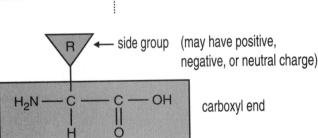

Figure 7.6
Structure of an amino acid

▶ MATERIALS NEEDED

For each pair of students:

- 3–4 extra-long pipe cleaners
- 1 set of 50 colored beads that can be threaded on the pipe cleaners
  - 10 red beads, representing positively charged amino acids
  - 10 green beads, representing negatively charged amino acids
  - 30 beads of a third color, representing neutral amino acids
- 1 container to hold beads
- 1 small geometrically shaped object such as a ball, a triangular block, or a cube
- cellophane tape

▶ PROCEDURE

NOTE: Many forces are involved in determining protein folding. For the purposes of this activity, you will consider only the attractive forces of amino acids (positive, negative, and neutral charges) in determining how a protein folds.

1. Join 3–4 long pipe cleaners together securely, end to end. Be sure that you can't tug them apart.

2. Thread the beads along the pipe cleaners in random order. The protein molecule model must be built of pipe cleaners (representing peptide bonds) and no fewer than 25 beads (representing amino acids).

3. Twist your protein molecule model around the three-dimensional object (the other molecule). In twisting your molecule two features are important:
   - The interaction of the protein molecule and the other molecule must show "specificity"—the binding molecule and the binding site must mirror one another; that is, they should match in shape and fit together in a lock-and-key fashion. A pocket or groove along the edge of the pipe cleaner should form, molding around the small object (such as a ball or triangular block) which represents the other molecule involved in the interaction. The goal is to make a space in the protein molecule into which the other molecule fits (relatively) precisely.
   - The protein molecule must be folded according to the principle of mutual attraction. Positively charged amino acids (red) will attract negatively charged amino acids (green). Neutral ones will have no effect on folding. In forming this pocket be sure to have two or three locations where red and green beads come together, as they might in a protein in which the folding is dependent in part on interactions between positively and negatively charged amino acids. This may require some squeezing or sliding of beads. You may wish to stabilize this "interaction" with pieces of cellophane tape.

4. In your notebook, draw a diagram of your model, indicating in words or drawings:
   - where the binding site is on your protein;
   - how the interacting molecule fits or binds at this site;
   - where the important interactions between the protein and the other molecule occur; and
   - how the structure of the protein defines the binding site.

5. Find a red bead that is important in forming the shape of the binding site, and substitute one green bead for it; also substitute a "neutral" bead for one red or green bead, which is important in forming the binding site. What happens to the shape of your protein? What happens to the shape of your binding site? Write responses in your notebook.

6. Remove (delete) a section of your protein. (You may cut the protein molecule, remove the cut piece, and rejoin cut ends if you wish.) Does this change the protein shape or binding site?

7. Write responses to the following Analysis questions and be prepared to discuss your model in class.

▶ ANALYSIS

1. Describe the factors that determine the shape of your protein model.

2. How have changes in the shape of your protein influenced the protein's ability to bind to your other "molecule"?

3. How does altering the shape of your protein change its function?

4. Describe the steps involved when the enzyme lactase breaks down lactose sugar into glucose and galactose. What would happen if the enzyme binding site were altered? What would be the consequences for the organism if this enzyme were altered?

5. Some molecules have more than one binding site. For example, RNA polymerase, the enzyme that copies the encoded message in the DNA into mRNA, has binding sites both for the DNA molecule and for RNA nucleotides. What would happen to the ability of this enzyme to carry out its function if one of the binding sites was altered or lost? What would be the consequences for the organism?

6. Based on what you know about the transfer of information from DNA to protein, how might a change in the amino acid sequence of your protein occur?

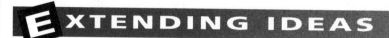

EXTENDING IDEAS

- Investigate diseases that are the result of changes in the sequence of a protein. Examples of this include sickle cell anemia, hemophilia, cystic fibrosis, Huntington's chorea, or lactose intolerance. Determine the symptoms of the disease, what protein is affected, what the function of that protein is (if it is known), what change has occurred to the protein, and how this is reflected in the DNA sequence (if it is known).

- Research how carbon monoxide poisoning occurs. What effect does carbon monoxide have on animals? How does it bring this effect about? Describe how this is an example of the principle, "another key that fits the lock." What does carbon monoxide do to the "lock?"

- A permanent wave is an example of the altering, or denaturing of proteins in hair. Explore the chemistry of a "perm."

ON THE JOB

PROTEIN CHEMIST   Did you know that no two proteins are alike? Protein chemists study the physical and chemical structures of proteins. Protein chemistry is one field of biochemistry, the study of the chemical reactions in living organisms and the effect of chemicals on life processes. Some protein chemists are involved in basic research which might involve isolating proteins by charge, mass, or shape, looking at their chemical structure and how each protein folds, or using the technique of crystallography to identify crystal structure which provides clues to the protein's function. Protein chemists involved in applied research might be involved in developing synthetic forms of proteins. Protein chemists work with chemical technicians in either a basic research laboratory or an applied research laboratory. Chemical technicians would look at the chemical content of a product, its purity, strength or stability or how to create new chemical products. This might include taking measurements, making calculations or collecting and analyzing data. A position as a chemical technician is available with a high school diploma or a two year college degree, as a laboratory assistant with a four year college degree. With a master's or doctoral degree chemists might be employed in supervisory positions in industry or pursue independent research in a university. Classes such as biology, chemistry, physics, algebra, geometry, foreign languages, English and computer science are recommended.

SCIENTIFIC ILLUSTRATOR   Are you intrigued by science, medicine and technology, but find your true passion to be drawing and illustration? Scientific illustrators combine their talent and technical ability in illustration with their scientific background to produce charts, graphs, illustrations or cover art for scientific articles and books. A scientific illustrator might be employed by a company or work as a freelance artist. Possible employers and clients are scientific laboratories in universities or in businesses, and publishers of magazines (both professional journals and those written for the general public), newspapers, and books. The illustrator's grasp of the subject matter is important in conferring with the doctors or scientists requesting the art work. Illustrations are created using computer graphics as well as by hand drawing. Some types of illustrations (such as medical illustrations) are better drawn by hand than by using the computer, because the artist is better able to portray the level of detail and complexity. Scientific illustration is a specialty of illustration and drawing because of its focus. Medical illustration is a specialty of scientific illustration. Medical illustrators enter special degree programs. In addition to taking computer graphics and drawing courses, they complete the first year of medical school, which includes anatomy classes and cadaver dissectionsp. Scientific illustrators usually have at least a four year college degree. Classes such as biology, chemistry, physics and other sciences, drawing, illustration, computer graphics, business courses, and English are recommended.

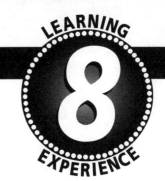

THE CHOLERA CONNECTION

PROLOGUE   **A** life without proteins would be no life at all—literally. In the last learning experience, you were introduced to the many and diverse functions that proteins carry out in living organisms. The functions of some proteins, such as certain enzymes and structural components, are well known; the functions of other proteins are not so well understood.

One of these little understood proteins is cholera toxin produced by the causative agent of cholera, *Vibrio cholerae*. What function this protein has for the bacteria is, as yet, unknown; however, its consequences for humans are all too clear in the symptoms of the disease it causes, cholera.

How does the presence of an infectious agent in a host cause disease? There is great diversity in diseases and the pathogenic agents that cause them, and a wide variety of mechanisms by which the symptoms of disease are produced. In this learning experience, you will investigate how one bacterial protein, cholera toxin, can cause the debilitating symptoms of disease. Based on your understandings of how the toxin affects cells, you will develop an approach to preventing the symptoms.

A DEBILITATING DISEASE

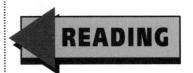
READING

Cholera is a serious disease that occurs periodically in epidemic proportions. In 1995, epidemics of cholera in South America, Africa, and eastern Europe caused at least 384,000 cases of the disease, resulting in about 11,000 deaths. Cholera is acquired by drinking water that has been contaminated with human feces or by eating food that has been washed in contaminated water.

V. cholerae, the bacteria that cause cholera, can be found in salt water or fresh water; they can also grow prolifically in human intestinal tracts. *V. cholerae* attach to the surface of the intestine and begin to divide. During this growth, the bacteria produce the protein, cholera toxin and secrete it into their immediate environment, the intestine, where it binds to proteins in the membranes of the intestinal cells. In normal cells, the flow of water molecules across the cell membranes is tightly controlled. The interaction of the toxin with the cell membrane *changes the structure of a protein in the cell membrane which regulates the flow of water in and out of the cell.* The result of this change is that water, salts, and other small molecules within the cell flow out into the intestinal lumen (passageway). This, in turn, causes the first main symptom of cholera—diarrhea.

A person with full-blown cholera can lose 20 liters of water daily because of copious diarrhea. Left untreated, patients rapidly become dehydrated, suffer from salt imbalances, and may die. One beneficial effect for the patient of this massive water loss is that it washes the bacteria out of the intestine. Thus, the disease can be cured spontaneously if the affected person can survive the acute phase of the disease. The most commonly used and effective treatment for cholera—fluid and salt replacement, also known as rehydration therapy—treats the symptoms of the disease and leaves the cure to the host's immune system.

To assume that *V. cholerae* bacteria produce their toxin for the sole purpose of harming their host would be assigning the bacteria human characteristics they do not possess (anthropomorphism). Why, then, do *V. cholerae* (or any bacteria for that matter) produce a protein that is toxic? One explanation is that the protein serves a survival function for the bacteria by inducing diarrhea. The diarrhea induced by this protein provides a kind of escape mechanism. This theory suggests that the human intestine serves as a rich environment for bacterial growth, providing an appropriate temperature and abundant nutrients, an incubator in which to multiply rapidly. The diarrhea provides the bacteria a means of escape and a return to the external environment where they can seek new hosts before the old host dies.

Another hypothesis suggests that the cholera toxin helps the bacteria obtain nutrients from damaged host cells by tapping into the energy, carbon, and other resources within the cell. By altering the properties of the membranes of intestinal cells, the toxin causes small molecules to leak out into the *extracellular* (outside the cell) environment where the bacteria live. This "permeability" of the cell membrane also causes the cells to lose water and salts and could cause the host to lose its life.

The explosive symptoms caused by cholera toxin may, in reality, be a kind of "mistake" on the part of the bacteria. In an ideal host/bacterial relationship, the uninvited guest would like to take up residence for as long as possible. As many long-term guests know, the best way to do that is to be unobtrusive. For *V. cholerae*, that would mean quietly colonizing the gut for a long-term stay without being too obvious about it. With this strategy it could continue to grow and reproduce, periodically passing its offspring out to seek new hosts. The devastating symptoms and mortality seen in many cases of cholera could reflect an unsuccessful attempt by the bacteria to colonize and a means of rapid escape when peaceful coexistence has failed.

Even though the culprit that causes cholera is known, and the mode of transmission is well understood, cholera continues to occur. The reason for this is simple: any conditions which foster crowding or poor sanitary standards can result in water contaminated with human fecal matter; this is a potential site of a cholera outbreak. Contaminated drinking water and unsanitary living conditions are facts of life in many areas of the world today, therefore, despite knowledge of the disease and its origins, cholera continues to be a serious public health problem.

▶ ANALYSIS

1. What roles do you think the toxin might play for the bacteria?

2. Not all *V. cholerae* bacteria produce a functional cholera toxin; certain mutants (both natural and laboratory-created) do not make a functional toxin. Do you think individuals infected with a mutant strain would display the symptoms of cholera? Why or why not?

3. Another model for the function of the cholera toxin in *V. cholerae* is that this protein enables the bacteria to stick around, literally. This model proposes that the toxin may serve as an adhesive, enabling the bacteria to form colonies on the inner surface of the host's intestinal lining. Recent investigations indicate mutants that do not make cholera toxin can colonize the intestinal lining just as efficiently as those that do make the protein. Do these results support or disprove the adhesive model? Explain your answer. How might these same mutants be used to prove or disprove the other models presented in the reading?

4. Using your understanding of information transfer in the cell and the importance of protein shape, propose a model (starting at the DNA level) explaining why the toxin in these mutants might no longer function.

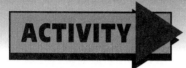

THE TOXIN TAKES A CELL

How does cholera toxin, the protein that gives cholera its characteristic of virulence, interact with the host cells? In the following activity, you will build a model of this interaction. Use available materials and your knowledge about how proteins interact with other molecules (based on your exploration in Learning Experience 7) to construct a model.

▶ MATERIALS NEEDED

For the class:

- assorted materials for constructing model proteins and their binding sites, such as: balloons, solution of salt water (1%), long pipe cleaners (chenille stems), colored beads, toothpicks, construction paper, gum drops, small marshmallows, grapes, etc.

▶ PROCEDURE

1. Prior to building the model, you should:
   - determine ways of showing how protein binding sites interact with other molecules;
   - determine a way to show how these interactions might alter the shape of the biomolecules involved.

2. Build your group model. As you work be sure to take into consideration the following points:
   - Proteins have a specific shape.
   - The cholera toxin protein and the protein on the surface of the cell interact with one another.
   - Each protein has one or more binding sites for substrates, and the shapes of the binding sites on the protein and substrates should "fit together."
   - Interactions of protein and substrate can cause a change in the shape of the protein or proteins; this change in shape results in some change in the components of the reaction.
   - This interaction alters the ability of the cell to maintain water and salt contents.

3. Present the model to the class. In your presentation be sure to indicate how:
   - the toxin interacts with components in the cell membrane;
   - the interaction affects each reacting biomolecule;
   - the interaction affects the cell;
   - the interaction produces the symptoms of cholera.

Cholera: A Grim Byproduct of Squalor

By Richard Saltus, *Boston Globe*, July 22, 1994

The dreaded news that cholera has begun a lethal rampage among starving masses of Rwandan refugees was no surprise to infectious disease specialists, who said yesterday that unless relief workers can restore some measure of sanitation to the crowded camps, the epidemic could spread indefinitely.

And cholera—a bacterial infection that causes diarrhea so severe that it can cause death in hours—may only be the beginning.

"We're concerned about a whole range of diseases: cholera, dysentery, food-borne illnesses, measles," said Robert Howard, a spokesman for the federal Centers for Disease Control and Prevention in Atlanta. "You have here a whole breakdown in sanitation and public health. This is potentially one of the largest-scale epidemic situations we have seen in many years."

With forecasts yesterday of up to 50,000 cases of cholera among the millions of Rwandans huddled in eastern Zaire, officials of the CDC's International Health Program were preparing to send not only doctors but also at least one engineer to the refugee zone to give advice on the enormous sanitation problem, Howard said.

Virtually unknown in industrialized countries, cholera is endemic in parts of Asia, Africa and the Middle East where poverty and inadequate sanitation expose people to water or food contaminated by human waste. The bacterium that causes it, known as *Vibrio cholerae*, can spread rapidly whenever the social order breaks down and masses of people crowd together, making sanitary disposal of wastes impossible. This is the case now in Zaire.

Once infection begins, a toxin produced by the bacterium in the small intestine triggers uncontrollable diarrhea that quickly depletes the body of water and vital minerals called electrolytes.

"The disease produces massive amounts of stool that contain the organism, and it can get into food and water," said Dr. Mary Wilson, an infectious disease specialist at Mount Auburn Hospital in Cambridge and the Harvard School of Public Health.

The huge influx of refugees from war-torn Rwanda into Zaire, with its few facilities for housing, health care or sanitation, "created an ideal environment" for diseases to spread rapidly once the organisms got a start, Wilson said. "One could predict that other food-borne diseases, like shigella, will become a problem, and measles also can be devastating, especially to children, in situations like this."

Continued on next page

Sometimes cholera causes only mild symptoms, but it can be so severe that "people can lose many gallons of water in a 24-hour period," said Dr. Leo Liu, a specialist in infectious disease at Harvard Medical School and Boston's Beth Israel Hospital.

Pregnant women, children and the elderly are especially prone to the life-threatening consequences of losing so much fluid. Untreated, victims become unbearably thirsty, stop producing urine, and suffer weakness and muscle cramps. Their circulatory system may simply collapse. Up to 50 percent mortality has occurred in some epidemics, though it can be as low as 1 percent if health care resources are available.

In large epidemics, Liu added, health workers place the weakest, sickest patients on "cholera cots"—canvas cots with a hole beneath the buttocks, so that the continuous outpouring of watery diarrhea can be caught in basins or cans. "You have to dispose of all this contaminated water, or the bacteria will just spread," Liu said.

Antibiotics can help rid the body of the cholera bug, but the mainstay of treatment is replacing fluids and salts in patients. If they can be "rehydrated" quickly, cholera patients generally recover in a few days with no long-term effects. How to do this now in Zaire is what the international relief effort must figure out.
(Reprinted courtesy of the *Boston Globe*)

▶ ANALYSIS

1. Compare the cholera epidemic in Rwanda with the cholera epidemic in London during the 1830s (see Learning Experience 1).
   - What are the differences in living situations?
   - What might have brought on the disease in each population?
   - How did each population deal with the disease?

2. Compare what was known about the disease during the London epidemic with what was known in Rwanda.
   - What was known about how to treat the victims? How was this information used?
   - What was known about how to halt the epidemic? How was this information used?

3. Explain why the treatments used in the 1994 epidemic were effective. Use the information in the reading "A Debilitating Disease" to support your response. Why were these treatments not used in the London epidemics?

DESIGN THAT DRUG

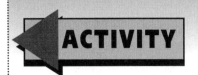

INTRODUCTION   You are a member of the scientific team of the "Drugs R Us" pharmaceutical company. Your company manufactures many designer drugs, chemical compounds that are specially designed for specific purposes. Once they knew how molecules interact with each other, scientists can design molecules that can compete for the binding sites used by infectious agents.

▶ TASK

1. Your current assignment is to develop a designer drug for cholera that will block the action of the cholera toxin. Be sure to take into consideration:
    - how proteins interact with each other;
    - how other biomolecules might be involved in these interactions;
    - how different biomolecules might compete for the same binding site.

2. As well as being a scientist in this company, you are also head of the Advertising Department ("Drugs R Us" is a very small company). Your next task is to design a full-page advertisement for a medical journal which describes your product. Be sure to include:
    - how the product is to be administered and why (orally, injected, in the water source, etc.);
    - what symptoms the product eases;
    - the biochemical basis for its activity;
    - how its effectiveness in treating the symptoms of cholera has been determined.

EXTENDING IDEAS

●   Toxins are also produced by other kinds of bacteria, including the bacteria of tetanus, *Bordetella pertussis*, and a pathogenic *Escherichia coli*. Research one of these pathogens. What is known about the mode of action of the toxin? How does it affect its host? What are the symptoms of the disease? Compare this with what you have learned about the cholera bacteria and cholera toxin.

●   Toxins from bacteria have been studied as part of different countries' programs in biological warfare. Research what toxin-producing bacteria have been considered for biological welfare, how these countries would use it, and how they would protect their own populations from the bacteria. Write an essay which speculates on the practicality and ethical considerations of countries developing such programs.

▶ One way of determining the effect of a drug on a disease is to test it on animals. Human testing of drugs and vaccines, called a clinical trial, is often carried out after the effectiveness and the potential side effects of the materials have been determined in animal models. Call your local hospital, university, drug companies, or branch of the Food and Drug Administration to determine whether any clinical trials are underway in your area. Find out what drugs are being tested, against what diseases, the protocol or way the trial is being conducted, and anticipated outcomes.

▶ Human experimentation has been a part of the history of scientific investigation in the United States. In some cases the course of a disease was followed in patients even though a cure was available. Investigate the Tuskegee experiments on syphilis in humans and prepare an essay on why this was done, what was learned, why the ethics of this approach have come under scrutiny, and what experimental alternatives might have been available.

▶ Infectious agents of plants also produce toxins. Some fungi that infect plants produce toxins called mycotoxins. When humans and other animals eat the plants, they may contract diseases, mycotoxicoses. One such disease is ergotism. Ergot is produced by a fungus, *Claviceps purpurea*, which infects rye and other grasses. Throughout recorded history, people have occasionally consumed fungus-infected rye, especially in times of famine when every last bit of grain was needed. The alkaloids produced by this fungus caused a wide range of devastating symptoms including memory loss, blindness, double vision, confusion, hallucinations, abortions, gangrene, and muscle spasms. In France the disease was called "sacred fire" because the afflicted individuals felt as though they were being burnt. Research ergot and its biological activity. Determine the impact of this disease economically and socially during the Middle Ages in Europe. Describe methods that are taken today to avoid this disease.

ON THE JOB

PHARMACOLOGIST   Have you ever wondered how your doctor knows how much medicine to prescribe? Pharmacologists conduct basic and applied medical and drug research to study the effects of drugs and chemicals in animals and humans. One area of pharmacology studies how the chemical structure of the substance interacts at the cellular and molecular level in organs and tissues. This research results in standardizing drug dosages and discovering how drugs can be used most effectively. Pharmacologists were involved in the development of anesthetics, antibiotics (such as penicillin), vaccines (such as tetanus and polio), tranquilizers, and vitamins. Pharmacologists may specialize in the effects of drugs on a particular part of the body such as the nervous system. In a second area of pharmacology, researchers study substances used in the environment, in agriculture, or in industry, and specifically study chemicals, food additives and preservatives, pollutants, poisons and other materials to determine their effects on humans. Pharmacology is a different career from pharmacy. Pharmacy is the health profession which prepares and dispenses drugs to patients. Pharmacologists have a Ph.D. in pharmacology from a medical school or school of pharmacy and may be medical doctors (MD) as well. Classes such as chemistry, biology, physiology, mathematics, computer science, physics, and English are necessary.

PUBLIC HEALTH NURSE   Are you interested in nursing, but not in working only in a hospital or in an office? Public health nurses or community health nurses are health care professionals who work with individuals and groups of people to promote health, prevent disease, and when needed care for the sick or injured. Public health nurses often travel from one community to another, compared with general-duty or office nurses who might work in a hospital or in another health care facility such as a physician's office, public health agency, school, camp or Health Maintenance Organization (HMO). Public health nurses have specialized training which allows them to practice many and varied nursing skills. For example, visiting patients who are at home rather than in the hospital might involve taking the patient's temperature, pulse or blood pressure, administering medication or injections, recording symptoms and progress of the patient, changing dressings, or assisting the patient with personal care. Visiting an expectant mother might involve helping the parents learn how to take care of newborns and how to feed and care for their babies. With additional training to expand skills and knowledge, registered nurses may become nurse practitioners and do many tasks previously handled by physicians (such as making diagnoses and recommending medications). There are several different program sequences that provide nursing training. With a two year program in nursing, it is possible to work in any of the settings described above. With a four year college degree in nursing it is possible to hold an administrative position or work for a public health agency. A master's degree makes it possible to become a clinical nursing specialist and focus in one field of nursing (for example, working with cancer patients or in a cardiovascular unit) or to teach in a school of nursing. In all cases, students must pass a licensing exam to become registered nurses and practice nursing. Classes in subjects such as biology, chemistry, mathematics, physics, and English are necessary.

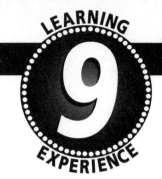
EMERGING DISEASES, EMERGING PROBLEMS

PROLOGUE **M**edical science has made tremendous advances against the scourges of infectious disease. Early in the twentieth century, predictions were commonly made that infectious diseases would soon be relegated to science history as public health measures and technology seemed to eliminate the problems globally.

These predictions, however, have not come true. Infectious diseases remain the major cause of death worldwide and a leading cause of illness and death in the United States. Since the early 1970s, appearances of diseases with symptoms never before described and diseases once thought vanquished have been routinely reported worldwide. Newly identified pathogens and their associated diseases have included the human immunodeficiency virus (HIV) which leads to AIDS, Legionnaires' Disease, hantavirus, Lyme Disease, hepatitis C virus, and toxic shock syndrome. Reemerging diseases (that is, diseases once thought under control but making a comeback on the public health scene) include tuberculosis, malaria, cholera, pneumococcal diseases, salmonellosis, and staphylococcal infections.

Figure 9.1
Examples of outbreaks of emerging diseases worldwide

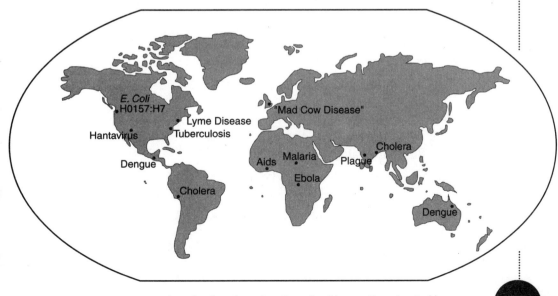

What are the origins of so-called new diseases that are reported in the news with increasing regularity? Are they really new diseases caused by new pathogens, or does a new set of circumstances enable a disease to appear in the population? Why are some diseases, once thought to have been conquered by modern medicine, reappearing in new, more virulent forms?

In this learning experience, you will begin a long-term research project in which you will investigate, in depth, the circumstances, biological and social, which can result in the emergence or reemergence of a disease.

READING

THEY'RE EVERYWHERE

Some of the diseases that have emerged and the social changes that enabled them to spread to new places are described below.

- AIDS is thought to have originated when a virus was trasmitted from African wild monkeys to humans by an as yet unknown mode of transmission.

- Lyme Disease is transferred from deer ticks to humans as the result of increased human contact with deer in suburban areas.

- Dengue fever was unknown in the United States until the virus's mosquito vector was transported accidentally from Asia in shiploads of tires filled with rainwater.

- In the 1960s, the Peace Corps set up pumps in many villages in Africa to bring water. These pumps also brought malaria by creating new breeding grounds (puddles of standing water) for the mosquito vector of the parasite.

- The building of the Aswan Dam in Egypt brought water for agriculture, but also brought epidemics of yellow fever, a viral disease, and schistosomiasis, a parasitic disease.

- Outbreaks of cholera continue to occur as people crowd into cities to find jobs or into refugee encampments to escape the ravages of war.

A change in either the virus itself or the vector which carries it may result in the emergence of a new disease or the reemergence of a known one such as the following examples.

- Canine parvovirus, which appeared in dogs in 1978 and causes life-threatening distemper, seems to have originated from a mutation in the feline parvovirus that enabled the virus to infect a new host.

- When first identified hantavirus caused kidney infections. A change in a viral protein appears to have altered the tissue specificity of the virus, resulting in a severe, often deadly, lung disease.

- Tuberculosis, gonorrhea, and staphylococcal infections, once considered almost vanquished, have increased because of the misuse of antibiotics and the development of drug-resistant strains of the bacteria.

- Misuse of insecticides also has resulted in the resurgence of disease; the development of insecticide resistance in the mosquito has resulted in the reappearance of malaria, once almost nonexistent in regions where insecticides were used.

Recent discoveries have begun to implicate infectious agents as the cause of diseases previously considered noninfectious, including:

- Bacteria of the species *Helicobacter pylori* have been well established as the causative agent of peptic ulcer disease.

- Human papillomavirus, which can be transmitted during sexual activity, is associated with cervical cancer in women.

- Hepatitis C virus is now considered the leading cause of chronic liver disease, cirrhosis of the liver, and has been associated with liver cancer.

- The sexually transmitted *Chlamydia trachomatis* bacteria have long been implicated in infertility, and another strain of *Chlamydia* has recently been associated with coronary artery disease.

- The infection in utero of a fetus by *Toxoplasma gondii*, a parasite, has been shown to cause congenital mental retardation.

EMERGING DISEASES

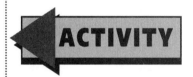

INTRODUCTION   In this module, you are exploring the nature of infectious diseases and the agents which cause them. In this long-term research project, you will need to apply the concepts from the module in order to understand the factors involved in the emergence or reemergence of a disease. At the end of the module you will present the findings of your research to the rest of the class as a public health policy that you have developed for creating strategies to reduce the risk of future outbreaks of this disease.

In preparation for the final presentation, you will be working in groups of four. Each group will be responsible for developing expertise about an emerging infectious disease. At this point you may not have all the background to address some of the issues. Some of this background will be acquired in the remainder of the module and some you will acquire through your own research.

▶ TASK

Work as a group, assigning responsibilities for efficiency. (However, all members of the group are responsible for knowing how to carry out each step and for knowing the information and group recommendations.)

1. Select the disease your group wishes to research, either from the list in the reading "Emerging and Reemerging Diseases" which begins on page 99 or another emerging or reemerging disease of your choice.

2. Gather resources on the epidemiology, environmental and social factors, and biological data of your diseases from the library, Internet, public health policy groups, local health professionals, and national organizations such as the Centers for Disease Control and Prevention (CDC) and the National Institutes of Allergies and Disease. When conducting research, look for information that will help you respond to the questions that follow.

- **EPIDEMIOLOGY**
    - When and where was this disease first recognized?
    - Why is this disease considered emerging or reemerging?
    - How many documented outbreaks have there been?
    - What are the mortality rates? (How many individuals have died?)
    - What are the morbidity rates? (How many individuals were made ill?)
    - What population has been affected by this disease?
    - What characteristics (habits, travel, work, relationships, gender, cultural practices, etc.) did this population share that may have contributed to the outbreak?
    - What methods were used to trace the outbreak?
    - Who has done the research? What is the story behind their research and investigation into the outbreak?

- **ENVIRONMENTAL AND SOCIAL FACTORS**
    - In what kind of environment did the pathogen first cause illness?
    - Describe the communities which have been affected. Did any social customs, economic factors, or political difficulties occur or change which might have provided the pathogen with a new host or might have facilitated the spread of the disease? If so, explain what happened and how these factors created an opportunity for the pathogen.
    - Did any changes occur in medical practices (such as changes in drug use, new procedures, loss of health care facilities, reduction in prevention programs)?

- Did any changes occur in the local or global environment (such as deforestation, reforestation, drought, famine, global warming) which might have caused new opportunities for the host/pathogen contact? If so, explain what happened and how these factors created an opportunity for the pathogen.

- **BIOLOGICAL DATA**
  - Describe the mode of transmission of the disease. How was this determined?
  - What is the nature (virus, bacteria, parasite) of the causative agent? How was this determined?
  - Describe what is known about the biology of the pathogen. Where in the host does it grow? What requirements does it have to maintain its own life functions? How does it affect the host's ability to maintain its life functions? Which biological functions in the host does the pathogen disrupt?
  - What characteristics of this pathogen enabled it to enter a new host?
  - What kind of immune response does this organism provoke in its host?
  - What are the symptoms it produces? What is the biological basis of these symptoms?
  - Is it related to other familiar or unfamiliar pathogens? Did any changes occur in the pathogen (such as changes in virulence, development of drug resistance, changes in tissue or host specificity) to cause this new or reemerging disease? If so, describe these changes and how they contributed to the appearance of this disease.

  Because not everything is known or understood about these infectious agents yet, you may not find the answers to all of these questions. If this is the case for your disease, explain in your presentation that certain data is unavailable, or has not yet been ascertained by the experts. Be aware that information about diseases and their agents changes continually, and today's "facts" are sometimes tomorrow's fiction due to new findings and discoveries in research.

3. Develop a public health policy.

   Once you have gathered your resources and information in the areas described above, you will be responsible for designing a public health policy which proposes strategies for reducing the risk of future outbreaks. This policy must consist of strategies that are realistic and take into account the context of local social conditions in which they are to be carried out, the living conditions, the economic status of the area, the political situation, and any changes which are occurring in the area. So, for example, do not propose a high-cost solution to problems in a desperately poor developing nation. Do not try to change centuries-old social customs and habits. Do gain a perspective of the culture and economic situation in which this disease is occurring.

Your policy should include the following:
- a brief description of the disease; its epidemiology, the nature of the causative agent, the events which led to the outbreak in the area;
- strategies for reducing the occurrence of this disease (such as developing programs for education in behaviors to reduce risk, implementing changes in sanitation infrastructure, expanding health care and public health services, developing vaccines or drugs, and developing programs to determine risks involved in certain environmental development programs). Include an explanation of why these strategies would be effective.
- methods for identifying and containing future outbreaks should they occur (surveillance systems for the early detection, tracking and control of the disease).

4. Prepare your presentation.

    The final presentation, which should last about 10 minutes, should include:
    - appropriate information and background materials on your disease;
    - a description of your public health policy, the rationale behind it, and an explanation of how it takes into account the specific social and economic conditions of the community in which the disease occurs.
    - Visual aids which help facilitate your presentation.

    The presentation will take place at the end of the module. At the close of each presentation, the teacher will ask follow-up questions, and then the class will discuss your public health policy proposal. Altogether, the presentation and follow-up discussion should take about 20 minutes.

5. Compare the emergence of different diseases.

    As you listen to other presentations, take notes on the following:
    - common themes that have been observed about emerging diseases;
    - how the problem of infectious diseases should be addressed in making public policy;
    - what strategies could be put in place for anticipating the rise of new diseases.

    A discussion at the end of the presentations will address these questions.

► EVALUATION

Your final presentation will serve as an assessment. The presentations will be evaluated by your teacher and fellow students on the following criteria:

– Have you gathered sufficient and appropriate information?

– Have you reached logical conclusions about your emerging or reemerging disease based on the information and ideas you have gathered?

– Does your presentation reflect insight and understanding of the reasons for emergence or reemergence of the disease?

– Does your public policy proposal demonstrate knowledge about local conditions at the site of the outbreak? A thoughtful and feasible response to those conditions? An understanding of the problems posed by the pathogen you have been studying?

– Is the presentation organized, clear, and effective? Does the presentation enable the audience to become engaged and interested in the topic?

– Are you able to respond concisely and clearly to questions from the audience?

– Does your presentation demonstrate that each member of your group has been involved in the process of researching the information, defining the policy, and preparing the presentation?

EMERGING AND REEMERGING DISEASES

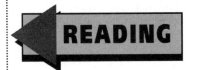

The following are some examples of diseases which have been classified by the CDC as emerging or reemerging infectious diseases; that is, diseases that have shown increased occurrence in humans within the past two decades. With your group read through the list and choose a disease which you would like to investigate. Alternatively, your group may select a disease of your own choosing but you must confirm that this disease is considered an emerging or reemerging disease.

ACQUIRED IMMUNE DEFICIENCY VIRUS (AIDS)

Caused by the Human Immunodeficiency Virus (HIV), AIDS was first recognized as a new and distinct clinical disease in 1981. Initially identified as a disease of homosexual men, AIDS has developed into an increasing threat to all populations. Transmitted by sexual contact or by blood contact, it is estimated that more than 22 million persons are currently infected with the virus with 8,000 new infections occurring everyday. Early infection with HIV shows no detectable symptoms, but its site of infection (white blood cells of the immune system) leaves infected individuals susceptible to a variety of rare and not-so-rare diseases. Since no cure or treatment is presently available, death is the inevitable outcome of infection. Death is generally caused by one of the diseases rather than directly by HIV.

HEMORRHAGIC FEVER

In 1976, a terrifying disease made its appearance in Zaire. Caused by the Ebola virus, this disease is characterized by massive internal bleeding and kills nine out of ten individuals infected. The disease reappeared in Zaire in 1995. Epidemics of this disease have resulted from transmission by direct contact with infected individuals or laboratory monkeys. The most recent epidemic in Zaire was believed to be spread by the funeral practices of the people. Ebola virus spreads through the blood and replicates in many organs, causing extensive damage which results in bleeding, shock, and death. No specific cure or vaccine exists.

LYME DISEASE

First described as a disease during an outbreak in Lyme, Connecticut, in 1975, Lyme disease is caused by spirochete bacteria that are transmitted by a tick vector. The disease is becoming a major problem in many parts of the United States, particularly in suburban areas where deer and human populations are living in closer proximity. The symptoms of Lyme Disease include swelling around the infected area and flu-like symptoms which, left untreated, can develop into neurologic and cardiac problems.

HEMORRHAGIC COLITIS (FAST-FOOD SYNDROME)

In 1993, children in the state of Washington were coming down with bloody diarrhea (hemorrhagic colitis). Subsequent reports of this disease have appeared in Minnesota, Massachusetts, and other states. The causative agent has been identified as *Escherichia coli* 0157:H7. Infection has most commonly been linked to eating undercooked beef such as hamburgers. Initially associated with foods served in fast-food restaurants, contaminated beef has begun to appear in supermarkets. The bacteria can also be transmitted through poor hygiene practices.

TUBERCULOSIS

Tuberculosis, also known as consumption and the great white plague, was one of the leading causes of death prior to the introduction of antibiotics in the 1940s. Between 1953 and 1984, the number of new cases of tuberculosis, which is caused by rod-shaped bacteria, dropped from 84,000 to 22,000. Public health workers foresaw the end of tuberculosis in the twenty-first century, but in 1985 the case rate began to increase at an alarming rate due to the appearance of multi-drug-resistant strains. Transmitted through droplets formed during coughing by infected individuals, the symptoms include fatigue, loss of weight and appetite, fever, and a persistent cough. If left untreated, death is common. A vaccine known as BCG confers some protection but is not readily available in the United States.

TOXIC-SHOCK-LIKE SYNDROME

Headlines such as "New Flesh-eating Bacteria Stalks Population" flashed across newspapers and tabloids in the early 1990s. Individuals who had suffered minor wounds or injuries were experiencing symptoms of severe invasive infections that were causing extensive damage to soft tissue and in many instances resulting in death. The infecting agent was identified as *Streptococcus pyogenes*, long known as the causative agent of a childhood disease, scarlet fever. Scarlet fever, which is characterized by a diffuse rash and fever, had been a common disease prior to the 1950s, when it virtually disappeared, most likely due to the use of penicillin to treat sore throats which are also caused by *S. pyogenes*. However, in recent times this pathogen appears to have returned with a vengeance, appearing first as a skin or wound infection and then developing into bloodstream infections sending the patient into shock.

MALARIA

Far from being a new disease, malaria has been known since antiquity. Caused by the parasitic protozoan *Plasmodium*, which is transported by a mosquito vector, malaria causes widespread disease and death in Africa and Asia. At various times in history, malaria was thought to be a conquered disease; eradication of the vector brought relief to the United States and many parts of Asia. But malaria is back. Misuse of antibiotics and insecticides has resulted in drug-resistant strains of the parasite and insecticide-resistant mosquitoes. Malaria is on the rise and the arsenal with which to combat it has diminished. Approximately 300 million of the world's people are afflicted with the disease, and each year between 1 to 1.5 million die, many of them children. Symptoms include fever, shivering, pain in the joints, and headache.

BOVINE SPONGIFORM ENCEPHALOPATHY ("MAD COW DISEASE")

Bovine Spongiform Encephalopathy (BSE) became a significant problem in Great Britain in the early 1990s when this neurological disease began affecting significant numbers of cattle. An alarm was sounded in the mid-1990s when several young men and women in Great Britain died of a rare, particularly in young people, neurological disease which affects the brain and spinal cord, causing sponge-like lesions. As these symptoms resembled those found in cattle infected with BSE, the question was raised as to whether the infectious agent (a somewhat mysterious agent called a prion which appears to be made up entirely of protein) could be transmitted by ingesting contaminated beef. The possibility of such an epidemic raised a serious threat both to the health of beef-eating individuals and to the British economy, which is dependent on the export of beef.

READING ➤

BEHOLD THE CONQUERING PATHOGEN

Despite all the technological and medical advances made in the twentieth century, today's physicians, policy-makers, and scientists sometimes find themselves in a position reminiscent of the one John Snow found himself in, back in 1854. In the last forty years, medical researchers and physicians have been confronted with unfamiliar, sometimes terrifying diseases.

In the following article, David Satcher, director of the CDC in Atlanta, describes some of the lessons and challenges that emerging and reemerging diseases present.

Excerpt from

Lessons and Challenges of Emerging and Reemerging Infectious Diseases

David Satcher, ASM News. vol. 62, No. 2, 1996.

In 1821....Americans had an average life span of well under 50 years, and the vast majority of deaths were due to infectious diseases. In the first half of the 19th century, problems such as malaria, yellow fever, and cholera were present even in the mid-Atlantic states, and respiratory diseases such as diphtheria, pneumonia, and rheumatic fever were the routine killers of children and adults. Even at the turn of this century, infectious diseases remained the leading cause of death, with tuberculosis leading the entire list in the United States.

Now that is no longer the case. Over the course of the 20th century we have made tremendous progress in our efforts to control infectious diseases. Perhaps the best-known accomplishment in this area is the eradication of smallpox, with the last case occurring in Somalia in 1977. Smallpox thus became the first disease in history to be completely eradicated from the world. As a result, millions of people around the planet will no longer needlessly suffer a painful death and disability from this dreaded disease.

Following on the heels of the smallpox success, polio is well on its way to eradication. Over a period of only 40 years, we have gone from a situation in which millions of children were stricken with this terrible disease every year to the recent certification of the western hemisphere as free of polio.

Major advances have also occurred on a number of other fronts; the number of measles cases in the United States reached a historic low in 1994, and *Haemophilus influenzae* type B disease is rapidly fading as a leading cause of childhood meningitis and sepsis as a result of the introduction of conjugate vaccines in the late 1980s.

These spectacular successes have occurred for a number of reasons, including improvements in the standard of living (including basic sanitation and hygienic measures), the development and introduction of vaccines, and the development and introduction of antibiotics.

These successes have taught us some important lessons. First, combating disease requires a strong collaborative effort between the basic sciences, clinical medicines, and public health. Polio provides an example: basic scientists developed vaccines to protect against disease; clinicians diagnosed disease, cared for patients, and delivered vaccines; and public health implemented vaccination campaigns and monitored for the occurrence of cases. None of these entities can perform alone and expect success. The second lesson is that when we put our minds to it, we can achieve spectacular results in the area of infectious disease control and prevention.

Not so many years ago, many of the best scientific and public policy minds in the country were ready to close the book on infectious diseases. Essentially we were victims of the very successes that I just mentioned. These experts believed that our vaccines and antibiotics would solve all of our problems and we could easily control any new problem that arose. As events of recent years have shown, these pronouncements were premature.

In the 1990s, infectious diseases account for more than 50% of deaths throughout the world, and we are increasingly faced with new and reemerging disease challenges. Examples of these threats include the worldwide AIDS epidemic, which is now 15 years old and growing; the resurgence of tuberculosis in the late 1980s; the new hantavirus first detected in the southwestern United States in 1993; the 1994 epidemic of plague in India; diphtheria sweeping across the former Soviet Union; a new cholera strain in south Asia; and the frightening reemergence, for the first time since 1979, of Ebola virus last year [1995] in Zaire.

Virtually every year brings information on a newly recognized pathogen, such as the herpes virus responsible for Kaposi's sarcoma and the morbillivirus which killed horses and their trainer in Australia. Compounding the problem, our microbial foes have developed an amazing capacity to resist our control efforts, particularly through the development of drug resistance, and we are helping them by injudiciously prescribing and taking antibiotics. Probably more than anything else, emerging antibiotic resistance threatens to reverse many of the hard-fought gains made in the control of infectious diseases in the last century.

Why is this happening? There are many factors responsible for the resurgence of infectious diseases, including human behaviors, and demographic changes, technologic and industrial advances, changes in the environment, international commerce and travel, and a breakdown of public health control measures.

LESSONS FROM EMERGING AND REEMERGING DISEASES

We have learned and are learning several lessons from emerging and reemerging disease. First, we must never take for granted the adaptability of the

Continued on next page

microbial and parasitic coinhabitants of this planet with whom we compete for space and resources, including food. Just as we have the ability to create new weapons such as vaccines and antibiotics and pesticides, these coinhabitants have demonstrated the ability to develop new defenses, new pathways, and new armamentaria [inventory of resources] for survival and growth. We see it in the drug-resistant *Streptococcus pneumoniae* organisms or the enterococci. We see it in the drug-resistant malaria that is now ravaging parts of Africa. This ability to survive, to change, and to grow is a major force of our coinhabitants that we cannot afford to underestimate.

Second, just as human behavior, demographics, and lifestyles have been shown to be major factors in chronic disease epidemiology, it is increasingly clear that they are major factors in emerging and reemerging infectious disease. Examples include antimicrobial misuse and resistance, the role of sexual behavior in AIDS transmission, the role of cooking practices in *Escherichia coli* O157:H7 transmission, the role of funeral practices in the spread of Ebola virus in Africa, and the role of human-rodent interaction in many parts of the world in supporting diseases such as the plague in India or the hantavirus in the southwest.

The third lesson is that progress in modern technology and changes in ecology and land use often bring with them unintended and undesirable consequences. Examples include the invasion of the rain forest in South America and Africa and the appearance of new viruses such as Bolivian hemorrhagic fever virus, Guanarito virus, and Ebola virus and air handling systems, and the emergence of Legionnaires' disease.

The fourth lesson is that increasingly we live in a global community and public health, in order to be effective, must be global in nature and outlook. We are today less than 24 h [hours] away from almost any community in the world, and people who encounter an infectious disease agent in one part of the world today may be in a totally different part of the world tomorrow. We must remember that viruses, bacteria, and parasites do not need visas to cross borders and they even occasionally ride first class.

The last lesson is that prevention of infectious diseases makes economic sense in addition to medical sense. A dose of measles vaccine saves $17 [for each dollar spent on treatment] in health-care expenses. Once polio is eradicated, it is estimated that the global savings will be >$1.5 billion per year. And in the mid-1980s we estimated it would take about $40 million in federal expenditures to eradicate tuberculosis from the United States. Now we are spending over $100 million annually as a result of its resurgence and the emergence of multiresistant forms. As is true of most medical problems, prevention of infectious disease pays.

If we keep these lessons from emerging infections in mind, they will serve us well in years ahead as we attempt to be a healthier people in a healthier world through prevention.

All of this change has contributed to the rising threat of infectious disease to the health, well-being, and perhaps even survival of the human population. Surprising as this threat may be, perhaps it is not unexpected. Joshua Lederberg, winner of the Nobel prize in Medicine in 1958, made the following statement:

> *It is still not comprehended widely that AIDS is a natural, almost predictable, phenomenon. It is not going to be a unique event. Pandemics are not acts of God but are built into the ecological relations between virus [bacteria, parasite], animal species, and the human species, and we had better understand that or we will rue it".*

> *Excerpted from J. Langone.*
> *"Emerging Viruses."* Discover
> Magazine, *December 1990.*

In this long-term project, you will have the opportunity to decide whether you agree with Dr. Lederberg's statement and what factors have come together to result in the emergence of the disease you are investigating.

▶ ANALYSIS

1. What do you think is meant by a "new or emerging disease"? Where might a "new disease" come from?

2. Describe some of the biological, social, political, and economic issues that might be involved in the emergence or reemergence of a disease.

3. Many social and economic endeavors have unintentionally resulted in the emergence of infectious diseases. For example, in the building of the Aswan dam, an unforeseen result was that it also assisted in epidemics of yellow fever and schistosomiasis. What do you think of this trade-off between agricultural progress and disease occurring in an area? Do you need more information in order to decide? If so, what kind of information will help you? Do you think that projects such as the Aswan Dam should take into consideration the possibilities of infectious disease which might be brought on? Why or why not? What information might be needed to predict such an outbreak?

4. What does Dr. Lederberg mean in saying we will "rue it" if we do not pay attention to the ecological relations between infectious agents, animals, and humans? Do you agree? Why or why not?

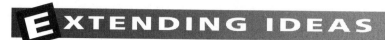

Chronic fatigue syndrome (CFS) is a disorder characterized by profound tiredness and weakness; patients with CFS become exhausted after mild physical exertion and are often unable to conduct the routine tasks of life with fatigue. A difficult illness to diagnose since incapacitating fatigue is associated with a wide range of well-defined diseases, CFS was officially given disease status in 1988. Most often occurring in white women between the ages of 25 and 45, the cause of the disease has not been determined. No evidence exists that CFS is communicable through person-to-person contact, or even that it is a communicable disease but several lines of research implicated the possible involvement of several well-characterized viruses. Research CFS, its clinical aspects and demographics and possible causes then decide whether you think it is an infectious disease. Support your decision with evidence from your research.

Viral Hitchhiker

PROLOGUE   **O**ften, sick people will say that they "caught a bug" or "picked up a germ" somewhere. No one with a runny nose or an upset stomach is likely to care whether the infection is bacterial, viral, or parasitic; they just want the symptoms to go away. In reality, though, there are huge differences among these organisms; and why you are getting sick is, in part, a reflection of these differences. As you have seen, bacteria can cause symptoms inadvertently with the byproducts of their metabolism. Viruses can cause symptoms, in part, because of their total dependence on the host's cellular machinery.

In the next three learning experiences, you will be investigating the effects of viruses on their hosts and how this can result in disease in the host.

Invasion of the Cell Snatchers

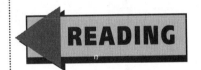

In the late 1800s, the tobacco crop in Russia was being destroyed by a disease that left the plants mottled and spotted; the leaves of afflicted plants looked like a mosaic of light- and dark-green areas. In 1892, a Russian biologist, Dimitri Ivanovsky, carried out experiments to determine the cause of the blight.

The existence of bacteria as causative agents of disease had already been determined by Louis Pasteur and Robert Koch. Pasteur had developed a technique for isolating bacteria and determining whether they were able to cause disease. He tested infectious fluids by passing them through a filter; if the material which was retained on the filter was able to cause infection and the filtrate (the liquid which passed through the filter) was not, the presence of a bacterial agent of infection in the original fluid was indicated.

Ivanovsky applied Pasteur's technique, using an infectious extract from tobacco plants suffering from the mottling disease. He found, to his surprise, that the filtrate, rather than the material retained on the filter, was fully infectious when applied to healthy plants (see Figure 10.1). As

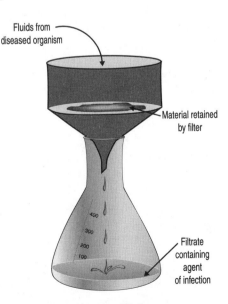

Fluids from
diseased organism

Material retained
by filter

Filtrate
containing
agent
of infection

Figure 10.1

the filtrate was able to satisfy Koch's Postulates (see Learning Experience 3), it must have contained an infectious agent. Up until this experiment, all known infectious agents were too large to pass through a filter. This observation led to the recognition of the existence of a whole new class of infectious agents, much smaller than any previously known organisms.

The actual nature of the causative agent remained a mystery until 1935 when advances in technology made it possible for an American biologist, Wendell Stanley, to isolate and identify the cause of the mottling disease. He squeezed the juice from 2,000 pounds of tobacco leaves and from this juice extracted a residue that could be purified to form pure needle-like crystals. When the crystalline form was dissolved and applied to tobacco leaves, it could cause disease. The particles were named tobacco mosaic virus (TMV). Later tests showed TMV to be rod-shaped particles composed of more than 2,000 identical protein molecules forming a coat around a core of RNA.

Many viruses have been identified since the discovery of TMV. Viruses come in a wide variety of shapes and sizes (see Figure 10.2). Most viruses are hundreds of times smaller than bacteria or eukaryotic cells. Viruses are essentially genetic material wrapped up in a protein. They lack the cellular machinery required to carry out the basic life

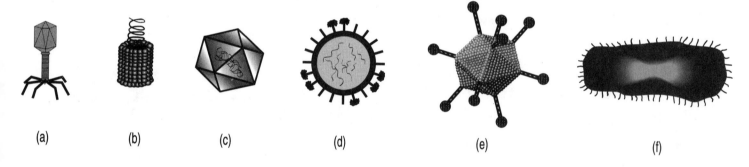

(a) (b) (c) (d) (e) (f)

Figure 10.2

Examples of various viruses: (a) T4 bacteriophage infects bacteria and contains DNA; (b) tobacco mosaic virus (TMV) infects plants and contains RNA; (c) poliovirus contains RNA and causes polio in humans; (d) influenza virus contains eight RNA segments and infects a variety of animals; (e) adenovirus is a DNA-containing virus which causes colds in humans; (f) vaccinia virus infects animals, contains DNA, and is a close relative of the smallpox virus.

processes for growth, reproduction, and response to stimuli: many viruses carry no enzymes to replicate their genetic material or transcribe nucleic acid into mRNA, and none have the protein synthesis machinery (ribosomes, tRNAs) to translate this information into protein. Viruses are inert until they enter a host cell and come to life by redirecting the host's cellular machinery to make multiple copies of the virus.

The genetic material of a virus can be either DNA or RNA. Viruses which have DNA as their genetic material include the causative agents of smallpox, chickenpox, and mononucleosis. Although we tend to think

Learning Experience 10   Viral Hitchhiker

of the genetic material as DNA, many viruses (such as poliovirus and influenza virus) have RNA as genetic material. Since the genetic material of a virus is generally small, it can encode only a small number of proteins. Generally, these proteins are those which make up the viral coat and enzymes which enable the virus to replicate themselves.

The proteins in the coat of the virus serve not only to protect the viral genetic material outside of the host cell, but also to assist viral entry to the cell. Each virus has a unique set of proteins which interact with surface molecules, usually proteins, on the membranes of the host cell. The viral proteins, like keys in a lock, enable the virus to gain entry into the host by binding to the host protein, or receptor.

In some cases, the proteins on the surface of the virus are very specific for binding and only permit the virus to infect certain types of plant, animal, or bacterial cells. For example, poliovirus will only infect human and monkey cells. In other cases, the viruses are able to infect a wide variety of cell types; influenza virus can infect humans, pigs, and ducks.

The following describes the steps involved in a viral infection. The steps are correlated to the numbers in Figure 10.3.

1. A virus must attach itself to an appropriate cell type.

2. The virus, or its genetic material, must enter the cell; if the whole virus enters, the protein coat must be removed to expose the genetic material;

3. The information in the viral genetic material must be read and translated into viral protein. These proteins may include enzymes specific for making more viral nucleic acid and viral enzymes (e.g., a viral DNA or RNA polymerase) and structural proteins used in assembling new viruses.

4. Many copies of viral nucleic acid must be made; anywhere from hundreds to thousands of copies are made in each infected cell.

5. Viral structural proteins must be assembled around each copy of nucleic acid forming a new virus.

6. The new viruses formed from the original infecting virus must be released from the infected cell to attack new cells and repeat this process. Viruses escape the cell either by bursting (*lysing*) the cell or by "budding" out of the cell membrane.

Figure 10.3
Steps involved in a viral infection

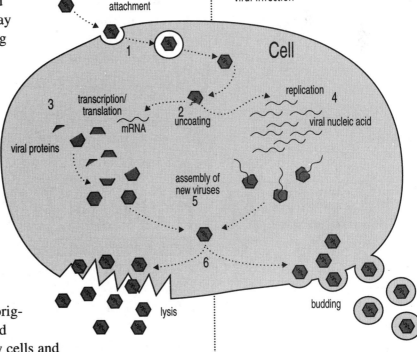

Until recently, viruses were thought to be the smallest infectious agent. However, during the 1980s an even smaller disease-causing agent, a *prion* was identified. The nature of prions remains very much of a mystery but they seem to be agents of deadly diseases of the central nervous system including Creutzfeldt-Jakob disease and Kuru, which cause dementia and death in humans, and bovine spongiform encephalopathy or "Mad Cow Disease" which appeared as an epidemic in cattle in Great Britain in the early 1990s. Surprisingly, prions seem to be entirely protein, with no detectable nucleic acid. How they infect, replicate, and cause disease is the subject of investigation in many laboratories.

▶ ANALYSIS

Write responses to the following questions in your notebook:

1. Why was Ivanovsky's discovery an unexpected result at that time? What was the significance of his discovery to the study of infectious disease?

2. In order to survive, all organisms must have the capacity to grow and reproduce. What are the difficulties confronting a virus in carrying out these life processes?

3. How does a virus make more of its nucleic acid and more protein? Where does it get the enzymes, cellular machinery, and building blocks to carry out these processes?

4. The proteins found in the coat of viruses interact with proteins on the surface of their host cell. Using your understanding of protein binding, describe how this interaction might make it possible for a virus to infect only certain kinds of cells. Use words and/or diagrams to explain.

5. Viruses are often referred to as "nonliving." Do you agree or disagree with this statement? Explain your answer.

ACTIVITY

A Pox [or TMV] upon Your Plant

INTRODUCTION What happens to a plant when it is infected by a virus? In fact, what happens when any organism is infected by a virus? Wendell Stanley dissolved the crystalline form of TMV, applied it to tobacco leaves, and found that it could cause disease. Tobacco mosaic virus (TMV), which is found worldwide, can infect more than 150 kinds of dicotyledonous plants (including tobacco, tomato, begonia, pea, bean, and petunia). The virus is very stable. It can survive in dried, infected plant material (such as cigarettes, cigars, and chewing tobacco) for many years. The symptoms caused by TMV can be either systemic or localized. In a *systemic* infection, plants have the mottled, mosaic effect observed by Ivanovsky; the leaves are a patchwork of light and dark green areas. In addition, the leaves are stunted in growth and parts of the plant may be distorted. These symptoms are caused when the viral infection spreads throughout the plant. In other kinds of plants, the infection may be *localized*; the virus remains at the site of infection in small necrotic lesions (areas of tissue breakdown). In a localized infection, the virus does not spread throughout the plant and none of the systemic symptoms are observed. In the following investigation, you will design an experiment to study infection in a plant.

▶ MATERIALS NEEDED

For each group of four students:
- 4 pairs of safety goggles
- 2 tobacco or tomato plants, 4–6 weeks old
- 2 pinto bean plants, 2–3 weeks old
- tobacco from several different brands of cigarettes
- 1 mortar and pestle
- 0.1 M (molar) dibasic potassium phosphate buffer, 10 mL
- 1 emery board file
- 2–4 cotton swabs
- 1 test tube
- 4 eyedroppers
- 1 graduated cylinder or pipette (5-10 mL)
- 1 small cup

For the class:
- additional dicotyledonous plants such as petunia, geranium, etc.
- monocotyledonous plants such as corn, different grasses, irises, etc.
- 500 mL distilled water
- access to a gram scale
- 1 graduated beaker or measuring cup (500-mL)
- access to a heat source
- soap or detergent
- 1 L (1 qt) household chlorine bleach
- spray bottles (atomizers)
- stock of pure tobacco mosaic virus (optional)

▶ PROCEDURE

1. Formulate a question regarding the disease-causing capacity of TMV, based on the readings from the module and on the following information, for your group to investigate:
    - TMV can be found in cigarettes; the amount may vary according to brand;

- TMV will infect certain kinds of plants but not others;
- TMV will cause one type of symptoms in some kinds of plants and other kinds of symptoms in different kinds of plants;
- TMV cannot enter plants directly through the leaf; if you wish to infect via the leaf, the leaf must be abraded (rubbed gently with an emery board).

Discuss with your group what you would like to find out about TMV in plants. Decide on one specific question you want to try to answer by conducting an experiment. Write down your question and discuss it with your teacher.

2. Propose a hypothesis based on what you know about viruses and infection, which might answer the question.

3. Design an experiment which would address this question and which you can carry out using materials from the materials list.

4. Outline the specific steps in the procedure that you will use in your experiment. Carefully think through the order in which you will carry out your experiment. You should take note of the following procedural techniques:

- If you are using tobacco from a cigarette, it will need to be ground into a slurry, or solution. Place two pinches of tobacco in the mortar. Measure in a graduated cylinder 5 mL of buffer. Then pour buffer into the mortar. Grind the mixture with the pestle until it is a fine slurry, and then use as needed in your experiment.

- When using the emery board on a leaf, gently abrade (scrape) the surface of each leaf you wish to infect. If you infect a plant in more than one location, note the position of each leaf on the plant and the age of the leaf. You may do this by sketching a picture in your notebook and labeling appropriately. *NOTE:* Do not scrape the leaf too hard. This will cause physical damage to the tissue.

- Use a cotton swab dipped in the slurry when infecting the abraded leaves of plants. After inoculating the leaves, gently rinse the leaves by running water over them using an eyedropper and distilled water. Be sure to have a cup under the leaf to catch the rinse water.

- Be sure to include a negative control (and a positive control if possible) in your experimental design.

5. As you design the experiment, indicate how you will collect and record the following data and observations:
- the appearance of the plant and leaves on any control plants;
- the appearance of the plant and leaves on the experimental (infected) plants;

- when symptoms of the disease first appeared on each plant;
- the severity of symptoms over the incubation period for each leaf;
- the total number of leaves infected and the degree of infection;
- how the experimental plants compared to one another in terms of symptoms;
- location of infection, rate of the appearance of symptoms, severity of symptoms; and
- any other differences or similarities that you have observed.

6. Show your procedure to your teacher before starting your experiment.

7. Collect materials for your group. Set up your experiment. Be sure to label your experimental and control plants clearly.

8. Place the plants in a sunny or well-lit area for 5–7 days. Observe your plants and record your observations every day. Set up a data chart to describe the condition of leaves and plants.

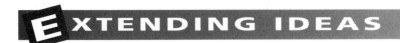

EXTENDING IDEAS

ON THE JOB

BOTANIST   Does the great variety of plants on Earth amaze you? Botanists are scientists who study all aspects of plants, including development and life processes, heredity, and anatomy. Plant science includes studying organisms such as algae, fungi, lichens, mosses, ferns, conifers, and flowering plants. The specialty within plant science that a botanist chooses can vary greatly. With an interest in ecology, botanists study the interactions of plants with other organisms and their environment. Field botanists travel the world searching for new species of plants or conduct experiments to discover how plants grow under different conditions. Botanists might study the whole plant, look at individual cells, try to identify how plants convert chemical compounds from one form into another, or conduct research to identify how the genetic information in DNA controls plant development. The research done by botanists is used to help develop new medicines, new foods, fibers, building materials or other plant products. Botanists work in a variety of places, such as botanical parks, forests, rangelands, wilderness areas, museums, industry, government laboratories or in universities. With a four year college degree positions as a laboratory technician or technical assistant are available. With a master's degree advanced research positions are available and with a doctoral degree it is possible to teach or do research in a university. Classes such as English, foreign languages, math, chemistry, physics, biology, and history are needed.

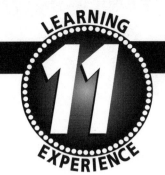

I Opened the Window and In-flew-enza

The title originates in a nursery rhyme:

> I had a little bird
> And its name was Enza.
> I opened the window
> And in-flew-enza

PROLOGUE **O**rganisms rarely live a singular, noninvaded existence. To paraphrase Jonathan Swift (Learning Experience 3), big organisms have little organisms; most living things serve as an environment for other living things. Some organisms can live together, one in or on the other, in perfect harmony (such as common intestinal bacteria), the invader producing no ill-effects in the host and even, at times, being beneficial. However, the life processes of other organisms, pathogens, can produce discomforting and sometimes fatal effects in their hosts. As you investigated in previous learning experiences, the toxin produced by the bacteria *Vibrio cholerae* provides some (as yet undefined) function for the bacteria. In carrying out this function for the bacteria, the toxin binds to a membrane protein in the intestinal cells of its host and causes the devastating symptoms of cholera. Other pathogenic bacteria and parasites may cause symptoms when their life processes interfere with a biological function of the host, deprive the host of vital nutrients, or cause structural damage to the host.

What, then, makes a virus pathogenic? Viruses lack the cellular machinery necessary for maintaining the characteristics of life. What happens when a virus enters the host organism? How is a virus able to make more of itself if it lacks all the necessary cellular machinery to carry out the life processes? What causes the symptoms of viral infection in a host?

An important approach to answering these questions employs a technique called polyacrylamide gel electrophoresis (PAGE). This technique enables scientists to analyze the protein content of a cell and determine the events that occur when a virus invades a cell. In this learning experience, you will be examining data generated by electrophoresis to determine what happens when a virus takes up residence in a cell.

READING

A Protein Guide to the Cell

A distinguishing characteristic of the identity and function of a cell is its protein content, or *protein complement*. The proteins in a cell determine what activities the cell can carry out. For example, a red blood cell must contain hemoglobin in order to transport oxygen; a muscle cell must have the proteins actin and myosin in order to be able to contract; a liver cell uses many proteins for getting rid of toxic substances in an organism's body (catalase is an example of one such protein). In addition, proteins in all of these cells enable them to carry out activities referred to as "housekeeping functions;" that is, necessary functions for maintaining life and carrying out the cellular processes of metabolism. All in all, a cell contains hundreds of different proteins.

If you wanted to examine which proteins a cell was making at any given time, how could you go about it? First, you would need to mark or label the proteins that are being made in some way to visualize them. Proteins in a cell can be labeled with radioactivity by using certain laboratory techniques. Cells are provided with radioactive amino acids which are incorporated into the cellular proteins as they are synthesized. Any proteins containing these amino acids will also be radioactive (see Figure 11.1). After the proteins of the cells are labeled in this way, the cell can be broken open or lysed by detergent to release the proteins and other biomolecules. (This is called a *cell extract.*)

The next step is to separate the proteins from one another in order to distinguish them. *Gel electrophoresis*, a method for separating biomolecules, depends on two physical properties: mass (or size) of the biomolecule and its overall (or net) electrical charge. The biomolecules to be analyzed are

Figure 11.1
(a) Molecules of methionine (a kind of amino acid) containing the radioactive element sulfur are added to media in which cells are growing. (b) The cells take up the amino acids and incorporate them into proteins being made on ribosomes.

a)

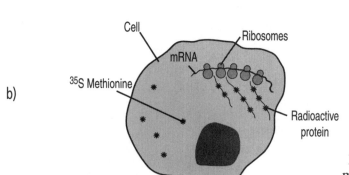

^{35}S Methionine

Media

Layer of cells

b)

Cell

mRNA

Ribosomes

^{35}S Methionine

Radioactive protein

placed in a gel matrix, and an electrical current is passed between a negative electrode at one end of the gel and a positive electrode at the other end. Many biomolecules have a net negative charge and therefore will move toward the positive electrode. The gel matrix itself acts as a sieve (much like a colander or strainer); it has pores of specific size which allow certain size molecules to pass freely but slow down the passage of larger molecules. The denser the matrix, the smaller the pore size, and the more the matrix retards the biomolecules' progress toward the positive electrode.

Many different kinds of biomolecules—most commonly, nucleic acids and proteins—can be separated (fractionated) by this technique. The ability to separate biomolecules in a gel matrix provides a way of analyzing the molecular components of cells, tissues, and organisms.

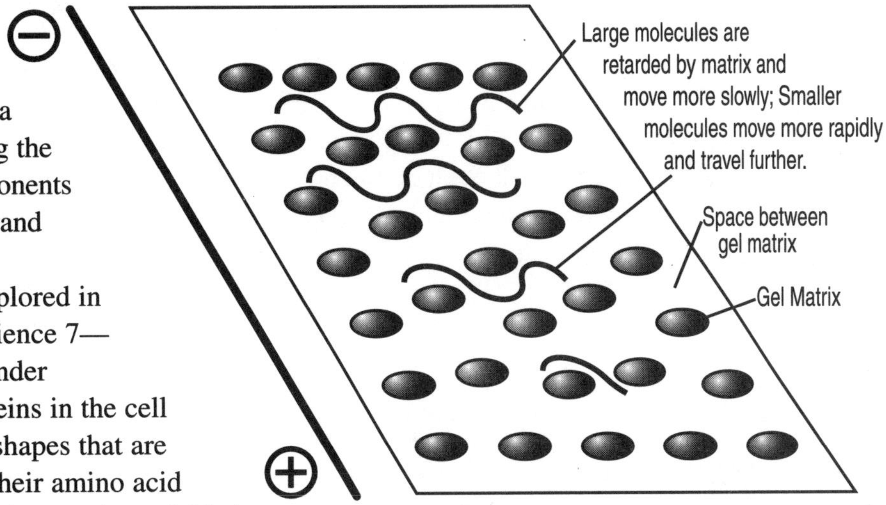

Large molecules are retarded by matrix and move more slowly; Smaller molecules move more rapidly and travel further.

Space between gel matrix

Gel Matrix

As you explored in Learning Experience 7—Protein, the Wonder Ingredient, proteins in the cell are folded into shapes that are determined by their amino acid sequences. Proteins can be unfolded or lose their shape in a process called *denaturation*. When you boil an egg, the albumin protein (white) of the egg becomes denatured and changes its physical characteristics dramatically. Heating a protein in a detergent also causes denaturation. In order to separate proteins by their true size, the proteins need to be unfolded. To do this, proteins are generally heated in a solution of a sodium dodecyl sulfate (SDS), an anionic (negatively charged) detergent that binds to most proteins. By binding to the protein, SDS has two effects: First, the detergent and heat interfere with the interactions that cause the folding in a protein; this disrupts the three-dimensional structure of the protein, causing it to assume a linear polypeptide chain shape. Second, the binding of the SDS masks any charge the protein may have (as a result of its amino acid content) by saturating the linear chain with its own negative charge. Figure 11.3 shows a protein in the presence of an anionic detergent.

Figure 11.2
Biomolecules of different sizes moving through a gel matrix

Figure 11.3
In the presence of SDS and heat, a compact folded protein (a) is denatured and (b) assumes a linear polypeptide chain structure because it is saturated with negative charges.

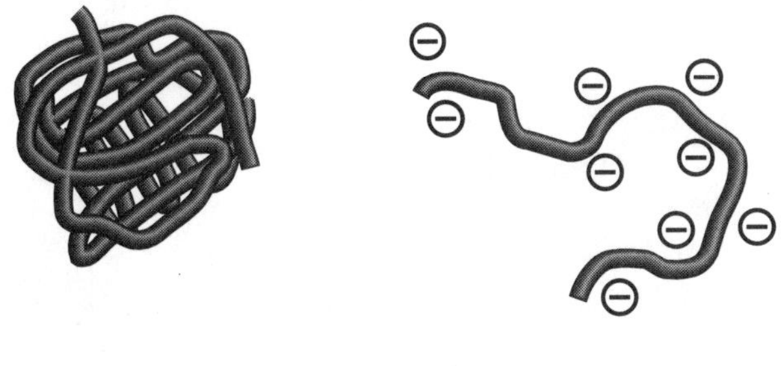

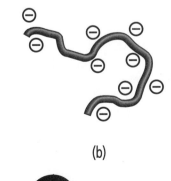

(a)   (b)

The basic procedure for analyzing the proteins in a cell involves the following steps, illustrated in Figure 11.4:

1. Cells are grown in a small culture dish in the presence of radioactive amino acids to label the proteins.
2. The cells are placed in a test tube and detergent is added to break them open and to release the cell extract; the extract may be heated to facilitate denaturation.
3. The cell extract is removed from the test tube with a pipette.
4. The extract is placed on top of a gel matrix and an electrical current is applied.
5. The proteins move through the matrix and are separated by size.
6. The proteins are visualized by exposing a photographic film to the matrix. When a film is exposed to radioactivity, the radioactivity causes the emulsion in the film to precipitate or come out of solution, much as when film is exposed to light.
7. When the film is developed, a black spot or band is seen wherever the film has been exposed to radioactivity. Therefore, wherever a radioactive protein is present in the gel matrix a corresponding black band will appear on the film.

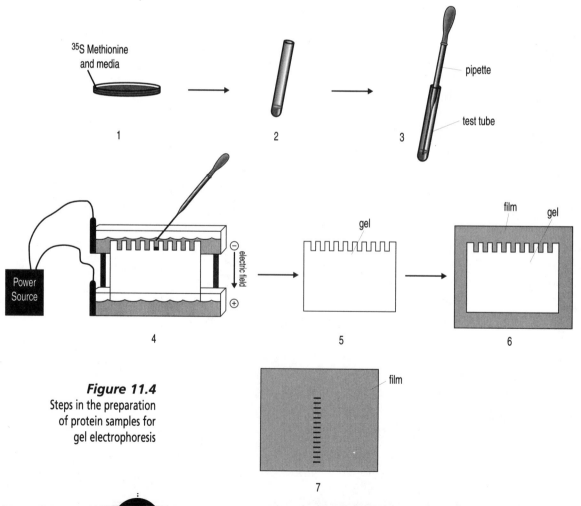

Figure 11.4
Steps in the preparation of protein samples for gel electrophoresis

ANALYSIS

Write responses to the following questions in your notebook in preparation for a class discussion.

1. What is the principle behind gel electrophoresis?

2. How might this technique help you if you were a physician with a patient whose red blood cells you suspected were not making the correct hemoglobin protein?

3. What can a research scientist learn by doing gel electrophoresis?

POP GOES THE CELL!

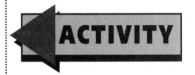

INTRODUCTION   In the following activity, you will simulate the process of polyacrylamide gel electrophoresis and examine the protein complements of two model cells, one of which has been infected with influenza virus.

MATERIALS NEEDED

For each group of four students:
- 2 paper bags representing two cells:
  - 1 normal healthy cell
  - 1 cell which has been infected by influenza virus

PROCEDURE

1. **STOP & THINK** Refer to "A Protein Guide to the Cell," and outline in your notebook the steps necessary to investigate the protein content of the "cells" you have been given. Explain the purpose of each step.

2. Using your desk or table top to represent the gel matrix, model the process of polyacrylamide gel electrophoresis on the paper bag cells.

ANALYSIS

1. Describe or draw your model of the separation of the proteins in your cell. Describe the protein content of each of your "cells".

2. What do you think the protein pattern indicates about the effects of influenza virus on the cellular processes of the host cell?

FLU WHO?

It has been said that viruses lie on the threshold of life, straddling the shadowy line between the living and the nonliving. Imagine that you want to take over a cell's resources and machinery so that the cell would be entirely devoted to your needs. How would you do it? The proteins encoded by the viral genetic material must be able to redirect the machinery of the cell toward the reproduction of the virus.

In order to investigate what happens to a cell and its proteins when a virus infects it, a scientist sets up two dishes of lung cell cultures. One dish contains only the nutrients (in a media) required by the cells for growth and radioactive amino acid; the other dish contains media, the radioactive amino acid, and influenza virus. As the cells grow, the radioactive amino acid is incorporated into the proteins being made. After 24 hours, the cells are removed from the dishes, placed in separate test tubes, and ruptured with detergent (SDS); the extract is then placed in separate wells (indentations) on top of a gel matrix. An electric current is passed through the matrix for several hours. After this time, the gel matrix is removed and photographic film is exposed to it for several days; the film is then developed.

► ANALYSIS

Examine the patterns from the gels in Figure 11.5 carefully and write responses to the following questions. Be prepared to discuss your responses in class.

1. What do the bands on the gels represent? What properties of the proteins caused them to separate in the observed patterns?

2. What differences do you observe in the patterns for the noninfected cell and the infected cell? What does the difference in the protein patterns tell you about what is happening in the infected cell?

3. Imagine you want to force a cell to make certain proteins in large quantities. Based on your understanding of viruses and the transfer of information in a cell from nucleic acid to protein, describe ways in which a virus might stop a host cell from synthesizing its own proteins and make only viral proteins.

4. Choose one of your ideas from question 3. Propose a model (that is, describe the steps involved) of what happens in a cell during such a viral infection. You may use words, drawings, diagrams, or a concept map.

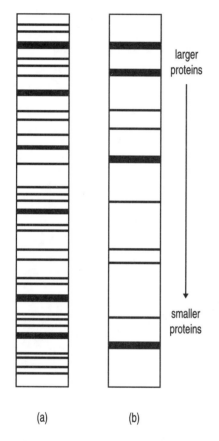

larger proteins

smaller proteins

(a)   (b)

Figure 11.5
Polyacrylamide gel analysis of (a) noninfected cells and (b) cells infected for 24 hours with influenza virus. Cells were grown in the presence of ^{35}S (sulfur-35) methionine, lysed in detergent (SDS), and fractionated on a polyacrylamide gel. After fractionation, the gel was exposed to film for five days. (The illustration is a diagrammatic representation of the results seen on the film.)

INFLUENZA: THE INSIDE STORY

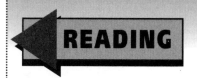

Let's look more closely at the influenza virus, commonly known as flu. Influenza travels from host to host through the air. Once flu enters the body through the gateways of the nose and mouth, attaches to receptors on the surface of the host cells in the lungs, and enters the cells, it releases its nucleic acid, consisting of eight pieces (segments) of RNA. Within the cell nuclei, these RNA segments are transcribed into mRNA. It is at this point that this virus might earn the name of "pirate." Influenza has evolved a very clever and efficient mechanism for commandeering the protein synthesis machinery of its host cell. In normal, noninfected cells, every mRNA has a sequence at one end called a "cap." This cap is required for the mRNA to bind to the ribosome and have its sequence translated into protein. Without the cap, no translation can occur. Influenza virus has evolved a mechanism for pirating the cap sequences from the host mRNAs and attaching them to its own messages. The result of this "pirating" is that the host mRNAs can no longer be translated but the viral messages can (see Figure 11.6).

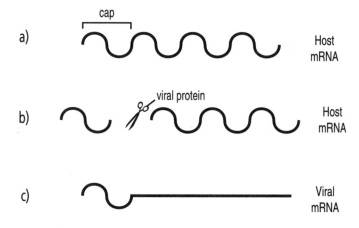

Figure 11.6
Virus stealing "caps" from host mRNA: (a) Host mRNA contains a sequence at one end of the molecule which is required for protein synthesis. (b) A viral protein cuts this sequence from the end of the host mRNA. (c) Sequence is attached to the end of the viral mRNA. The host mRNA can no longer be translated into protein, but the viral mRNA can.

The viral nucleic acid then proceeds to direct the synthesis of enzymes and proteins required for the virus to reproduce itself. The eight segments of viral RNA encode 10 proteins, 8 of which are found in the virus itself, and two of which are enzymes used in making the new virus. The virus proteins and nucleic acids are then assembled into virus particles that exit the cell by a process of budding; during the infection process two proteins, which are part of the final viral particle, are inserted into the host cell membrane. As the virus escapes from the cell it is encased in a lipid protein coat containing these two viral proteins which are embedded in lipids from the host membrane.

As RNA is less stable than DNA, RNA viruses are 100 times as likely to mutate or change their sequence as DNA viruses are. Within any group of RNA viruses are a large number of mutants. Most of them do not survive because they have no particular selective advantage over the unchanged virus. But, if the environment changes, some of the mutants may have an advantage. This genetic flexibility enables RNA viruses to move into new environmental niches, new geographical locations, and new populations. One potential result when the RNA virus mutates is that proteins making up the viral coat may alter; this change in coat protein may result in the virus being able to infect a new kind of host or evade the immune response of its normal host. (see Figure 11.7).

Figure 11.7
(a) Influenza RNA sequence mutates; (b) the change in sequence results in a change in one of the coat proteins. The * represents a change in one nucleotide.

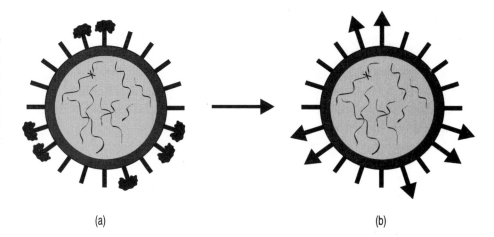

(a)   (b)

Influenza virus has an additional evolutionary advantage over most other RNA viruses. Its genetic material consists of eight very loosely connected pieces (or segments) of RNA. Influenza virus has a broad host range; that is, most flu viruses can infect a wide range of animals including humans, pigs, and ducks. When two influenza viruses from different animals enter the same host, segments of viruses of both types can mingle. For example, when a virus from a human infects a pig that is already infected with a pig influenza virus, the animal can serve as a mixing vessel for the creation of a new and deadly (to humans) influenza virus. The human virus may pick a viral segment of the RNA genome from the pig virus that encodes a completely different set of viral-coat proteins. The result would be as if the human virus took off its cloth coat and put on a pigskin leather jacket. (See Figure 11.8 on the following page.)

This kind of exchange can result in the emergence of a very new and different virus which is part pig virus and part human virus. This kind of event occurs rarely, only about once in every 10–40 years. But when it does, the ramifications for the human population can be severe. The flu pandemic of 1918 which killed 20 million people was the result of one such occurrence.

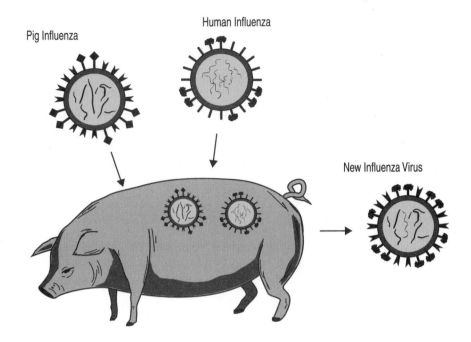

Pig Influenza

Human Influenza

New Influenza Virus

Figure 11.8
Infection of a pig with a pig influenza virus and a human influenza virus can result in a new type of influenza virus.

▶ **ANALYSIS**

1. Using the information provided in this reading, redesign the model you created in Question 4 from "Flu Who?" to reflect your understanding of the steps involved when influenza virus takes over the host cell. Include in your explanation how this model is supported by the data you analyzed.

2. Using your understanding of information transfer from DNA to protein, describe at least three other ways a virus might redirect a cell toward making its own viral proteins.

3. Describe how you think influenza virus might spread from an infected cell to a noninfected cell in the lungs.

4. Describe an experiment you could carry out, using the technique of polyacrylamide gel electrophoresis, to investigate the events involved in the infection of a cell by tobacco mosaic virus.

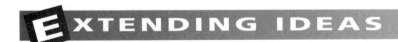

EXTENDING IDEAS

ON THE JOB

PUBLIC HEALTH EDUCATOR   Are you interested in working with a community to promote health and prevent disease? Public health educators work with individuals and the general public to work towards both promoting health and preventing disease within the population. These educators use specific methods, skills and program strategies to help individuals make behavior changes which encourage a healthier lifestyle, to learn how to use health services and to be aware of preventative measures that can protect against disease. Public health educators increase public awareness around issues such as cardiovascular disease, HIV/AIDS and sexually transmitted diseases, drugs and alcohol abuse, environmental hazards, unintentional injuries, health of expectant women and their children, and social violence. Public health educators work in a variety of settings such as community health centers, family and youth centers, elementary and high schools, advocacy organizations, and within a specific industry. Public health educators have either a master's or doctoral degree from a school of public health. Classes such as biology, chemistry, health, English, foreign languages, and computer science are recommended.

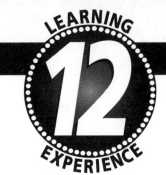

RETURN TO VIRAL HITCHHIKER

WHAT IS THE DIAGNOSIS?

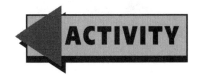

INTRODUCTION What are the effects of TMV on plants? In this learning experience, you will analyze the results of your experiment "A Pox (or TMV) upon Your Plant." Read the following Task section. You will need to write a final laboratory report and use the report for preparing a presentation.

▶ TASK

1. With your group, analyze your data. Discuss the meaning of the results and the conclusions that you can draw from them. (Be sure to take notes on the group discussion to use in writing your laboratory report.)

2. Plan your presentation. The presentation should include:
   – the project title
   – the names of research group members
   – the question that your group asked
   – a clearly summarized procedure
   – the data clearly presented, including graphs or tables where appropriate, and at least one diagram (a series of diagrams depicting changes observed is preferable)
   – a summary of your conclusions
   – the most significant information that you wish to share with other groups
   – any unanswered questions, new questions, and at least three suggestions for further study

   Include in your planning individual responsibility for preparing any illustrations, graphs, and text to be used in the presentation.

3. Write your own individual report which should include:
- the question being asked
- the hypothesis
- the design of the experiment
- the procedure
- the data and observations
- the conclusions from the data
- a discussion of whether the data answered the question and if not, why not
- any sources of possible error
- any new questions that came up as a result of this experiment

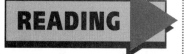

TO THE EATER OF THE SPOILED, BELONGS THE DISEASE

Salmonella are medically important bacteria that are responsible for two different diseases in humans. These bacteria are transmitted by improper handling procedures during food preparation and/or poor sanitation. One species, *Salmonella typhimurium*, causes a self-limiting, localized infection and is one of the most common causes of food-borne infections. When a human ingests this pathogen in contaminated food or water, a localized infection results in the gastrointestinal tract of the unlucky diner. Symptoms of food poisoning include nausea, vomiting, localized lesions in the intestine, abdominal pain, and diarrhea. Symptoms usually appear six to twenty-four hours after ingestion of the contaminated food and may last from a day to a week.

Salmonella typhi, on the other hand, causes an invasive, systemic infection, typhoid fever. The bacteria enter the bloodstream through the intestine and spread throughout the body. After multiplying in the spleen and liver, they are released back into the bloodstream. The symptoms of the disease include high fever, a flushed appearance and anorexia, sometimes accompanied by chills, convulsions, and delirium. If left untreated, typhoid fever can be fatal.

Why does *S. typhimurium* remain as a localized infection and *S. typhi* invade the intestinal wall and enter the blood stream to become a systemic disease? The answer is not known at this time, but the most virulent *S. typhi* strains produce a polysaccharide capsule. What role this capsule plays in the ability of the bacteria to invade systemically remains to be determined.

Interestingly, when mice are infected with *S. typhimurium*, the species that causes a localized infection in humans, it causes a systemic infection in the mice that resembles typhoid fever in humans. In contrast, *S. typhi*, which causes typhoid fever in humans, does not even infect mice.

▶ ANALYSIS

In a short essay, using diagrams or tables where helpful, compare localized and systemic infections of different hosts and different strains as exemplified by the diseases caused by tobacco mosaic virus and *Salmonella*. In your discussion include the importance of the identity of the host and of the infecting agent in determining whether the disease will be systemic or localized.

EXTENDING IDEAS

◉ In some people, *Salmonella typhi* hides out in the gallbladder, and these people can shed bacteria in their feces for years without showing any symptoms of the disease. Such chronic carriers cause major public health problems, especially when they are employed as food handlers.

The classic case of a chronic carrier occurred in the early 1900s. By tracing a number of typhoid cases back to their probable source, health officials first identified Mary Mallon, a professional cook in New York City, as a carrier who had caused several outbreaks and who came to be known as "Typhoid Mary." She was offered a gallbladder operation as a way of eliminating the source of the bacteria. (Antibiotics had not yet been discovered, so an operation was the only feasible solution to resolving her carrier state.) When she refused the operation, she was imprisoned for three years. She was then released, after promising not to cook for others. Apparently she did not take the allegations about her carrier state very seriously, because she changed her name and resumed her profession as a cook. She was subsequently employed by hotels, restaurants, and hospitals and managed to spread typhoid fever to many more people before she was finally apprehended. After her second apprehension, she was imprisoned again, this time for 23 years, until her death in 1938.

The identification and quarantine of individuals infected with contagious diseases has led to much discussion and controversy. Individuals applying for marriage licenses are required to undergo blood tests for syphilis. Legislation has been proposed barring immigration by individuals known to carry the Human Immunodeficiency Virus (HIV), the causative agent of AIDS.

Outbreaks of pneumonic plague in 1994 led to restrictions on international travel in and out of India. In an essay, discuss the moral and legal implications of such identification of and restrictions on individuals carrying contagious diseases.

▶ *Salmonella has served many purposes. It has been used as a model organism for studying bacterial metabolism and genetics and bacterial virulence. As a major cause of food-borne disease, it serves as an indicator of how safe a country's food and water supplies are. It is also the basis for many of the new oral vaccines. And now, believe it or not, someone has come up with a new use for* Salmonella—*as a means for honoring an admired public figure. Shortly after Michael Jordan announced his intended retirement from basketball, Dr. Stanford Shulman, Chief of Infectious Diseases at a Chicago, Illinois hospital revealed to the press that he was naming a new strain of* Salmonella *after Michael Jordan:* Salmonella mjordan. *We will probably never know whether Michael Jordan, in his heart of hearts, felt honored or otherwise by having a strain of diarrhea-causing bacteria named after him (would you?). One wonders how Mr. Jordan will represent this honor in his trophy room (if he has one), and how it will be handled by the Basketball Hall of Fame. Just keep it far away from the snack bar, guys.*

> Bacterial Pathogensis: A Molecular Approach, *by Abigail A. Salyers and Dixie D. Whitt, ASM Press, 1994, page 230.*

Describe how you might react if you were being honored by having a form of some dread disease named after you. Why would you react this way?

▶ Diseases of plants have profoundly impacted human lives. When crops that normally sustain populations are destroyed by epidemics of disease, famines are often the result. In 1733, 12,000 people on an island in Japan perished when rice stunt, a viral disease of rice, destroyed the crop. A fungal blight of potatoes in 1845 and 1846 decimated this primary staple food of the Irish people, causing a million deaths and mass emigration of 1.5 million individuals, many of them to the United States. In 1942 a fungal disease of rice in Bengal caused the deaths of 2 million people. Research one of these famines or another famine caused by a plant disease. Describe the characteristics of the infectious agent, the effect on the plants, and the social and economic ramifications of the disease on the population.

▶ Humans and other animals may be the victims of several degenerative disorders of the central nervous system, which appear to be caused by "proteinaceous infectious particles," or prions. Though these particles appear to be completely devoid of nucleic acid, they can cause transmissible diseases. The diseased state seems to be the result of a change in a normal cell protein. Research prions and describe what is known about how these infectious agents might be transmitted and how they can cause disease. *(For a review article, see "The Prion Diseases" by Stanley B. Prusiner,* Scientific American, *January, 1995. pages 48–57.)*

ON THE JOB

PATHOLOGIST   Are you interested in looking at how disease causes changes in organisms? Pathologists are scientists who study the diseases of plants and animals. Pathology includes identifying the agents which cause the disease, the interaction between the causative agent and the host, and the consequences of this interaction. Changes in the morphology and the function of cells are studied as evidence of changes in the health of the organism. Pathologists do both basic biomedical research, to identify the fundamental mechanisms of the disease process, and clinical medical research which includes diagnosing the cause of disease. The basic biomedical research includes studying normal and diseased cells and tissue at the cellular and molecular levels. Clinical research includes examining tissue samples from the skin, organs, blood or sputum and providing physicians with a diagnosis, or performing autopsies to identify the cause of death. The laboratory techniques and procedures used by pathologists are not unique to pathology, but are the techniques and tools used by chemists, molecular biologists and cell biologists. With a high school diploma or an associate's degree, positions as a laboratory technician are available. With a four year college degree, positions as laboratory assistants or research pathologists are possible. With a master's or doctoral degree pathologists can teach in a university or pursue independent research in a university or a laboratory. Classes such as biology, chemistry, anatomy, physiology, math, English, and computer science are needed.

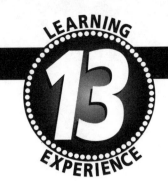
Immune System to the Rescue

The world we live in teems with microbial life. Every breath we take, every inch of our skin, every bite of food that enters our mouths, every surface we touch is covered with an enormous array of microscopic organisms. The majority of these microbes pose no threat. But a small number of these life forms—pathogens—can cause disease. Do we have any way to defend ourselves against these potential biological hazards in our environment? How is it that we usually stay healthy when agents of disease seem omnipresent? In this learning experience, you will explore some of the components of the *immune system*, the body's intricate and extraordinarily efficient defense against disease. The immune system is a diverse collection of specialized cells, organs, and structures designed to identify and destroy invaders before they destroy the host. You will model several events that occur when this system is confronted with pathogenic organisms.

The Pathogens Are Coming!

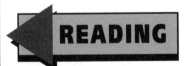

The body's first defense against pathogens is simply to try to keep them out. The skin, for example, acts as a physical barrier to the pathogens. It also carries out chemical warfare against infection by secreting oils and sweat which acidify the surface of the skin, making it difficult for potential pathogens to grow. Openings in the skin, such as the mouth and nostrils, provide easy portals of entry for infectious agents. These entryways into the body are protected by a modified type of skin called a *mucous membrane*. Not only can the mucous linings of these passageways physically trap microbes and debris, but some also contain anti-microbial enzymes which can break down or digest microorganisms. (see Figure 13.1)

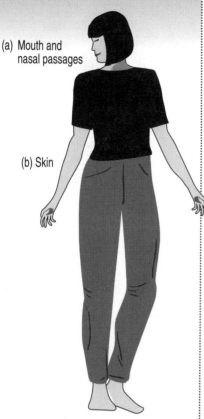

(a) Mouth and
nasal passages

(b) Skin

Figure 13.1
The body's first lines of defense against infection: (a) Openings such as the mouth and nasal passages are lined with mucous membrane which can trap microbes or actually destroy them with enzymes; (b) the skin provides a physical barrier and secretes oils and sweat which rinse the surface clean of microorganisms.

When microorganisms manage to get past the first line of defense, your body activates another set of defenses. Once invaders enter the body and find their target tissues (for example, lung cells, epithelial cells, intestinal cells), they begin their confrontation with components of the immune system. The immune system comprises many specialized cells that work in a cooperative effort of ordered reactions to recognize and defend the body against foreign invaders.

The immune response relies on proteins and their interactions. As you have seen throughout this module, proteins play many essential roles in maintaining life and in the recognition and communication processes which enable the immune system to stop an invasion.

Cells, bacteria, viruses, and parasites all have proteins on their surfaces. Just as you recognize your friends and relatives by their physical characteristics, your immune system recognizes substances as friends or foes by these proteins, a type of "identity card." In human cells, these proteins, called *major histocompatibility complex* (MHC) markers, enable the immune system to recognize "self" from "non-self" and make it unlikely to attack proteins of its own body. As you saw in Learning Experiences 7 and 8, the shape of a protein determines its function or activity. In this case, the shape of the protein marker tells the immune system if the shape is foreign or one of its own. If the shape is foreign, the immune system goes into action. Proteins synthesized by specialized cells of the immune system are sent out into the body through the circulatory system, acting as a call to arms for other cells of the immune system to initiate actions which help to defend the body. The circulatory system and the lymphatic system enable components of the immune system to travel to wherever they are needed in the body.

Molecules recognized by the immune system as foreign are called *antigens*. They may be carbohydrates and proteins on viruses, bacteria or parasites, pollen particles, or proteins inserted into the cell membrane during infection. In response to these antigens, other proteins called antibodies are produced by cells of the immune system. As you will see in this learning experience, these antibodies provide powerful protection against infection. The response of the immune system is dependent upon the specific interactions among cells and proteins; these specific interactions enable the immune system to recognize what does not belong and to take action to eliminate it.

▶ ANALYSIS

In your notebook, list the components of the immune system. (Include components in this reading and any others that you know about.) Next to the component write what you think it does as part of this system.

THE COMPETITION

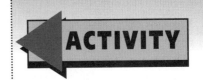

INTRODUCTION In many ways, the immune system is like a security system. It sends out alarms and keeps you well protected when something potentially harmful enters. To get a sense of how this line of defense works, you will design a security system of your own.

Imagine that you are the owner of an enormous corporation, Worldwide Communications. Your company has been extremely successful and is the envy of many other similar companies. Worldwide Communications is housed in a 700,000 square-foot building in a busy part of town.

Just recently, your research and development department created a stunning new invention: Your company is on the brink of establishing an innovative, wireless telephone system that will allow users to communicate by phone for a fraction of the costs they now incur. As a consequence, you have had a number of problems with attempts by your competitors to sabotage your equipment and steal your designs.

You are afraid that the security measures you have taken are not adequate. You and your team are meeting to try to solve this problem before it is too late. As part of your brainstorming strategy you need to define the problem and come up with some solutions.

► TASK

1. Identify ways in which your competitors could get into your building.
2. Identify ways they might gain access to your secret files.
3. Create a plan for protecting your corporation against the possibilities you identified.
4. Prepare a list of job descriptions for your security team.
5. Describe how these efforts will work together and back up one another to ensure tight protection against invasion.

CONFRONTATION!

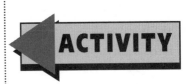

INTRODUCTION The immune system has two responses—cell-mediated and humoral—which work together to quell invasions of pathogens. You will need to determine how the components of the immune system work together to defend against infection by viruses. You will be using descriptions of immune system components and diagrams of the cell-mediated and humoral responses to determine how the immune system works. You will begin by exploring each component of the immune system.

▶ PLAYER OF THE IMMUNE SYSTEM	ROLE: WHAT IT DOES	WHAT IT INTERACTS WITH
MACROPHAGE 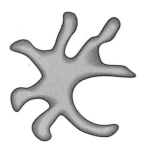	• Found circulating in the blood. • When a macrophage encounters a foreign antigen (a protein from a foreign invader) it engulfs viruses, bacteria, infected cells or cell remnants that display the antigen on the surface. • Macrophages display the engulfed viral antigen (protein) on their own surfaces by inserting viral antigen to its own cell membrane. • When a macrophage engulfs a virus, it calls other immune cells to the scene (termed the *cell-mediated response*). • When macrophages that have engulfed invaders encounter helper T cells; the T cells bind to the viral antigen on the macrophage surface. • When helper T cells bind to the antigen, the macrophage releases a protein called interleukin, an activating factor, which stimulates helper T cells to divide. • Macrophages engulf viruses, bacteria, or infected cells coated in the antibody.	• viruses • bacteria • an infected host cell displaying viral antigen on its surface • a cell remnant displaying viral antigen on its surface • helper T cells • viruses, bacteria, or infected cells with antibodies bound to antigens
HELPER T CELL 	• Originates in bone marrow, matures in thymus gland (thus the "T" in T cell). • Found circulating in blood. • First to arrive at infection scene when macrophages send out alarm. • Has protein receptors on its surface that distinguish foreign substances, bacteria, and viruses by the proteins found on their surfaces. • Recognizes viral and bacterial antigens on macrophage's surface. • Binds to viral and bacterial antigens on a macrophage, causing macrophage to release a chemical substance interleukin, which stimulates helper T cells to divide. • Releases activating factor, interleukin, which stimulates T cells and B cells to divide and activates killer T cells. • Part of cell-mediated response.	• macrophages • killer T cells • B cells
KILLER T CELL 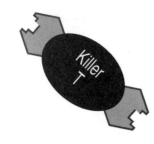	• Originates in bone marrow, matures in thymus gland (thus the "T" in T cell). • Found in circulating blood. • Can attack and destroy cells infected with active virus displaying viral antigens on their surface, by injecting toxic chemicals into them. • Part of cell-mediated response; arrives at infection when macrophages send out signal. • Activated by interleukin released from helper T cells.	• infected host cell displaying antigen on its surface

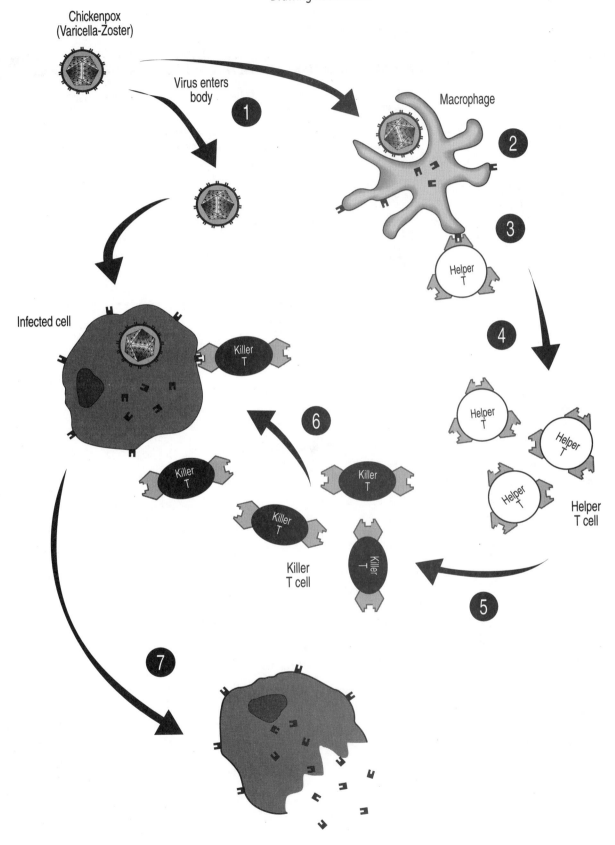

Figure 13.2

CELL-MEDIATED RESPONSE

Drawing not to scale

Chickenpox
(Varicella-Zoster)

Virus enters body

1

Macrophage

2

3

Helper T

4

Infected cell

Killer T

6

Helper T

Helper T

Helper T

Helper T cell

Killer T

Killer T

Killer T

Killer T

Killer T cell

Killer T

5

7

Table 13.3
Components of the Humoral Response (see corresponding Figure 13.3)

PLAYER OF THE IMMUNE SYSTEM	ROLE: WHAT IT DOES	WHAT IT INTERACTS WITH
B CELL	• Found in bloodstream, originates in bone marrow (thus the "B" in B cell). • May bind to viruses or bacteria using receptors on the B cell's surface called antibodies which recognize a specific antigen. • May bind with viral fragments found on infected cell surface. • B cells begin secreting antibodies that recognize viral and bacterial antigens. • Interleukin molecules, released from activated T cells, stimulate B cells to divide.	• viruses • bacteria • host cell with viral antigens displayed on its surface
ANTIBODY	• Produced by B cells. • Is a protein that has a precise recognition of an individual antigen. • Binds to viruses, preventing viruses from infecting cells. • Binds to viral antigens on the surface of infected host cells and tags those cells for destruction. • Macrophages engulf viruses, bacteria, and cells with antigens that have antibodies bound to them.	• viruses • bacteria • antigens on infected cells
MEMORY B CELL	• A B cell activated by interactions with antigens differentiates into a memory cell. • Remains after infection. • Ready to respond rapidly should the body ever encounter the same antigen again. If identical viruses or bacteria invade the body later, the antibody on the memory B cell binds to the viruses or bacteria and marks them for destruction. The virus is halted before infection is established.	• viruses and bacteria that have infected the body before

Figure 13.3
HUMORAL RESPONSE
Drawing not to scale

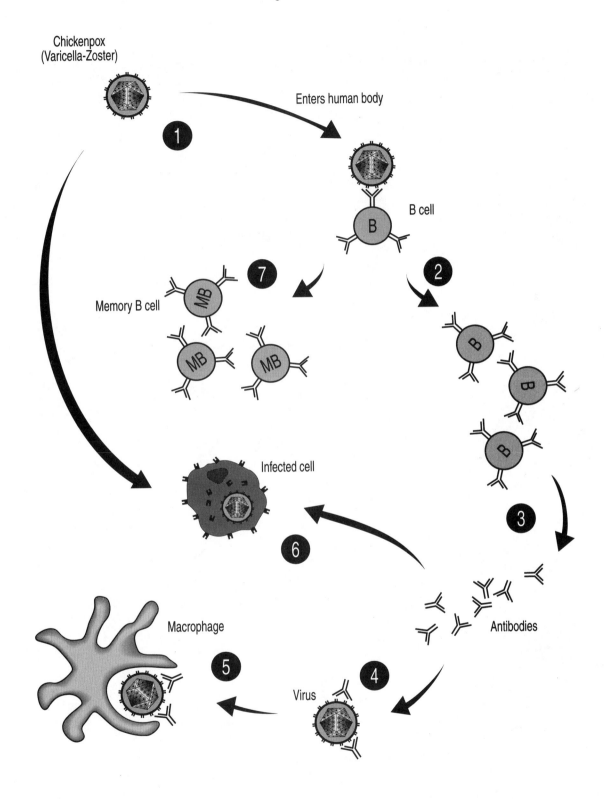

Chickenpox
(Varicella-Zoster)

Enters human body

B cell

Memory B cell

Infected cell

Macrophage

Antibodies

Virus

Table 13.4

Characteristics of Viral Invaders

INVADER	WHAT IT DOES

CHICKENPOX VIRUS 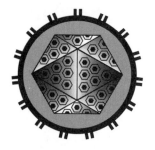	• May infect a host cell. Viral antigens are inserted into the cell membrane. The shape of the antigen expressed is unique.
	  – viral DNA, which codes for viral proteins, is injected into the host cell
	  – cell begins making viral proteins instead of cell proteins; DNA is replicated
	  – these proteins and DNA assemble into new viruses
	  – cell is disabled or killed and hundreds to thousands of new viruses are released
	• May be ingested by a macrophage.
	• May bind to memory B cell which has receptors that recognize specific *chicken-pox* antigens.

INFLUENZA VIRUS 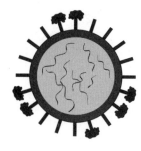	• May infect a host cell. Viral antigens are inserted into the cell membrane. The shape of the antigen expressed is unique.
	  – viral RNA, which codes for viral proteins, is injected into the host cell
	  – cell begins making viral proteins instead of cell proteins; RNA is replicated
	  – these proteins and RNA assemble into new viruses
	  – hundreds to thousands of new viruses are released by budding; cell dies
	• May be ingested by a macrophage.
	• May bind to a memory B cell which has receptors that recognize specific *influenza* antigens.

HUMAN IMMUNODEFI-CIENCY VIRUS (HIV) 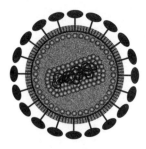	• Infects helper T cells.
	  – binds to receptor molecule on the surface of the T cell
	  – genetic material (RNA) is taken into the cell
	  – makes viral RNA and proteins which are assembled in virus particles
	  – virus particles bud out of the T cell and enter the bloodstream
	  – kills host T cell in the process
	• May also infect macrophages without being destroyed. Can grow and reproduce slowly without killing the macrophage.

Table 13.4
RESPONDING TO INFECTION BY CHICKENPOX
Drawing not to scale

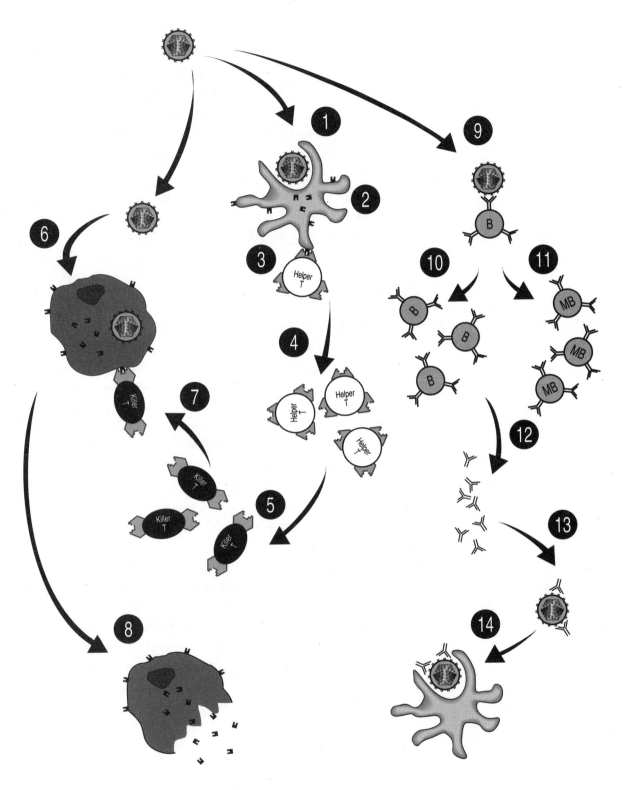

► CHALLENGES

Respond to the following in your notebook. Use the information in Figure 13.2 and 13.3 and Tables 13.2–13.4 in guiding your responses.

1. The body is infected with chickenpox virus. Write the steps of the immune response. (Use Figure 13.4 as a guide.)

2. The body is now reexposed to chickenpox virus. Write the steps of the immune response. Include a labeled diagram of the process.

3. The body has been infected with HIV. Write the steps of the immune response. Include a labeled diagram of the process.

4. While fighting chickenpox virus (for the first time), the body is infected with influenza virus. Write the steps involved in the immune response to this double invasion. Include a labeled diagram of the process.

► ANALYSIS

Write responses to the following in your notebook. Draw a diagram to help illustrate each response.

1. What would happen if a person were infected by a chickenpox virus but had no macrophages? If mounting an effective antibody response takes five to seven days, and the virus needs two to three days to establish a thriving infection, what are the possible outcomes for a person with this deficiency?

2. Why do people get chickenpox just once, but get flu again and again?

3. How do you think Griffith's encapsulated bacteria (Learning Experience 4—Search for the Cause) might have eluded the mouse immune system?

4. Acquired Immune Deficiency Syndrome (AIDS) is the disease associated with Human Immunodeficiency Virus (HIV) infection. Many people with AIDS suffer from opportunistic infections, that is, infections from organisms that their bodies could normally fight off. Explain how you think this might happen.

5. Based on your understanding of the immune response, speculate as to why the symptoms of HIV infection—AIDS—may appear many years after the initial infection.

WHY YOU FEEL CRUMMY WHEN YOU'RE SICK

by Robert M. Sapolsky, Discover Magazine, *July, 1990, pages 66–70.*

Recently, in preparation for a trip to the tropics, I received a dreadful number of inoculations. As I sat in the clinic after the shots, shifting from cheek to cheek in discomfort, the nurse explained that the vaccines—especially the one for typhoid—could make me feel a bit ill. And, sure enough, by nightfall I felt crummy.

It was a particularly unpleasant bout, because somehow it felt illegitimate. I wasn't really ill. I didn't have to worry that I had malaria or the flu or the plague. I knew what the cause was, and it wasn't serious. Vaccines, in essence, work because they fool the body into thinking it's just a little bit sick and had better defend itself. We're generally unaware of the mock battle being staged, but some vaccines, including typhoid shots, produce an unusually strong effect. So I couldn't really feel sorry for myself, and besides, I knew I'd be fine in the morning. In an odd way it was all form and no content—I felt sick without actually being sick.

An extraordinary array of illnesses make us feel crummy in this way. Mostly we just want to sleep. Our joints ache, and we feel cold and feverish. Sex loses its appeal. We lose interest in food; if the illness persists, we lose weight even if we force ourselves to eat. And we look like hell. Not long ago Benjamin Hart, a veterinarian at the University of California at Davis, listed 60-odd common diseases in mammals that produce the same array of symptoms, despite their infecting different organs. Give a person influenza, which affects the respiratory system, give a cat infectious anemia, which affects its blood, give a sheep enterotoxemia, which affects its gut, and all will get achy and mopey and feel like putting on flannel pajamas.

Traditionally, such symptoms were not considered terribly interesting from a medical standpoint. Suppose you had the flu and complained to your doctor that, in addition, you felt weak and your joints ached. I'd wager that the most common answer would be, "Of course you feel weak. Of course your joints ache. You're sick." The symptoms are so nonspecific and ubiquitous that they seem almost not to count. But in recent years researchers have discovered a great deal about why we feel crummy when we have infectious diseases. These symptoms don't just happen; a quite complex system of responses brings them about—and, it seems, for very sound reasons.

At the center of this story is the immune system and the various white blood cells it employs to fight off disease. When a pathogen—an infectious bug such as a virus or bacterium—invades the body, it is the immune system that first sounds the alarm: the invader is promptly grabbed by a large scavenger cell called a macrophage. The macrophage in turn presents the bug to a helper T cell, which signals that the noxious foreigner is indeed worth getting excited about. The macrophage then sets off a chain of events culminating in the activation of killer T cells that attack the intruder. This cascade is referred to as cell-mediated immunity.

Meanwhile, a second form of defense, known as humoral immunity, is also set in motion: the helper T cells stimulate yet another type of white blood cell—B cells—to divide, differentiate, and ultimately produce antibodies to the intruder. These in turn will grab hold of the infectious organism and immobilize it.

Sorting out this process has kept immunologists off the streets for decades. What they've learned is that the immune response involves a variety of cell types scattered throughout the body. To communicate with far-flung members, the immune system uses

Continued on next page

cytokines, chemical messengers that travel in the bloodstream and lymph fluid. And that's where feeling crummy begins to come in the picture.

Among the best known of these messengers are the interferons, which activate a type of white blood cell that fights viruses and cancer, and the interleukins, which are central to the T cell cascade. The inter-

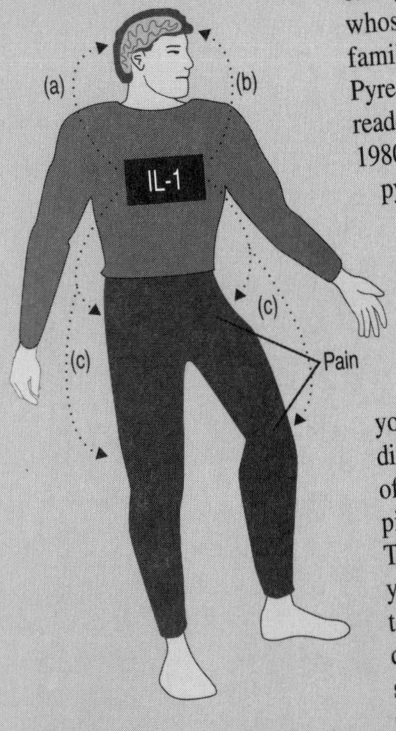

Figure 13.5
IL-1 causes many of the symptoms of disease. It (a) raises the temperature setting in the brain, causing body temperature to increase; (b) stimulates CRF production in the brain, reducing the appetite; (c) excites neurons in the nerve pathways, giving that achy, breaky feeling to every inch of the body.

leukin of greatest interest to us here is called IL-1; its principal job is to carry the alarm message from the macrophage (where it

is made) to the T cells. But we begin to feel crummy because that is not all that IL-1 can do; it can also influence the brain.

Most dramatically, this interleukin alters temperature regulation. For years it was known that, after infection, the immune system produced something that caused fever. No one knew what it was, and the putative messenger was called endogenous pyrogen, a term whose derivation should be familiar to pyromaniacs and Pyrex manufacturers among the readership. Not until the early 1980s was IL-1 identified as the pyrogen.

A part of our brain called the hypothalamus functions much like a thermostat. Normally it is set for 98.6 degrees. If body temperature drops below that, you shiver to generate heat, divert blood from the periphery of your body to vital organs, and pile on the blankets. Temperatures above 98.6 cause you to sweat and breathe faster to dissipate heat. What IL-1 does is cause the set point to shift upward. In other words, you begin to feel cold at 98.6, the various warming responses kick in and a new equilibrium is reached at a higher temperature. You are now running a fever.

But that's not the only way IL-1 makes us feel crummy. A few years ago two research groups (my own and a group in Europe) simultaneously reported that the chemical also causes the hypothalamus to release a substance called corticotropin-releasing factor, or CRF. This substance runs the

body's hormonal response to stress by initiating a cascade of signals going from the hypothalamus to the pituitary gland, and from there to the adrenal glands, which prepare you for an emergency.

Suppose you walk into the supermarket and, unexpectedly, find yourself being chased by a rhinoceros intent on goring you. You will start secreting CRF within seconds—and for good reason. CRF blocks energy storage: it inhibits the process by which the body stores fat as triglycerides and sugar as glycogen. Instead, energy is diverted in a hurry to the muscles that are hurtling you down the produce aisle. At the same time, CRF dampens appetite, sexual drive, and reproductive processes. These effects are particularly logical; this would be a foolish time to waste energy by ovulating or planning lunch.

And it is much the same during an infection. IL-1 triggers CRF release, and soon enough neither sex nor food seems particularly appetizing. Levels of sex hormones plummet, and if the illness lasts long enough, then ovulation and sperm production can be disrupted.

More crummy symptoms can be attributed to IL-1. It makes you sleepy—although no one is quite sure how—and it explains why everything aches.

There are nerve pathways coming from various outposts in your body—from the surface of your skin to deep within your muscles and tendons—that carry pain messages to your spinal cord; these messages are then relayed to the brain, which interprets them as painful. Obviously, stepping on a tack is a very painful stimulus: the pathway originating in your toe is going to be activated, and your brain will register pain in an instant. But far more subtle stimuli will not cross a pathway's activation threshold. They will not be perceived as pain unless the threshold is lowered. And that's exactly what IL-1 does; it makes the neurons along the pathway more excitable, inclined to react to things they would normally ignore. Suddenly, your joints hurt, old injuries ache again, your eyeballs throb.

Altogether, that's quite an impressive array of effects for a chemical that was once thought of only as an immune-system messenger. . .

One major aspect of the sick syndrome still needs to be explained: cachexia, or the wasting away of body weight. This is an obvious thing to happen during a sustained illness, given what happens to your appetite. But cachexia defines something more. During a chronic illness you lose weight even faster than can be explained by decreased eating. Your body has trouble storing energy.

CRF appears to account for some of that. Recall your desperate flight from the rhino in the supermarket: during such an emergency you need energy for your muscles at that instant, not later, and CRF, as we saw, indirectly blocks energy storage. But CRF also causes stored

energy to be released, returning fuel in the form of fat and sugar to the bloodstream. Thanks to IL-1 and hormones such as CRF, the same thing happens during an infection; if it goes on long enough, you lose your fat stores and begin to waste away.

But cachexia is also caused much more directly. When a noxious agent is first spotted in the body, macrophages secrete a second cytokine along with IL-1. In addition to its role as an immune-system messenger, this cytokine blocks the ability of fat cells to store fat. Reasonably enough, this chemical has been dubbed cachectin.

Looking at such a wide range of effects, it seems difficult to argue that feeling crummy is something that just happens for no good reason. Clearly, the body works very actively to bring those symptoms about. Various brain regions have evolved receptors for IL-1, and fat cells have developed specific mechanisms for responding to cachectin. There has to be some logic behind the evolution of these nonspecific responses.

Some of the symptoms make sense. A showdown with a virulent pathogen can require as much energy as a showdown with a rhino. It is no small task to trigger the massive proliferation of immune cells needed to mount a defense against infection: cells must divide and migrate at a tremendous rate, cytokines and antibodies must be hurriedly synthesized and secreted. All this immune activ-

ity does not come cheap; it requires a great deal of instant energy. Thus it is quite helpful for CRF and cachectin to block energy storage and keep fuel readily available.

It is also quite logical to inhibit reproduction if you're sick, since producing offspring is one of the most expensive things you can ever attempt with your body, especially if you are female—you're better off using the energy to fight the disease. If the disease is going to be around for a while, it is a particularly inauspicious time to get pregnant anyway.

By the same logic, it is probably a good idea to sleep more during an illness, because sleeping conserves energy. And maybe your joints hurt during a fever to make you conserve energy also—I'm not inclined to run around a lot when I ache all over. But it's unclear why you should lose your appetite, especially since many features of feeling crummy seem geared toward meeting the need for energy...

The most dramatic feature of feeling crummy, of course, is fever. The energy mobilized during an infection goes to fueling not only the immune system but the shivering muscles as well. During a malarial fever, for example, metabolism increases by nearly 50 percent, and much of this energy expenditure goes toward generating heat. An investment on this scale certainly suggests fever is doing something useful for you. And indeed a number of studies support the idea.

Continued on next page

The easiest way to demonstrate the benefits of feverishness would be to infect laboratory animals with something that typically causes a fever and see how they fare when the fever is blocked. You might, for example, administer an antipyretic drug such as aspirin and then monitor what happens to the animals' immune response, antibody concentrations in the bloodstream, and survivorship. If those measures are worsened, you can conclude that the fever normally helps fight the infection. . .

The reasons for this are at least two-fold. First, the immune system works better when you are running a fever. Studies show that T cells multiply more readily and antibody production is stepped up. Second, a fever puts many pathogens at a disadvantage. A wide variety of viruses and bacteria multiply most efficiently at temperatures below 98.6 degrees. But as a fever is induced, their doubling time slows. In some cases the pathogens stop dividing entirely.

Such studies suggest that fever and the host of other changes we suffer are adaptive mechanisms for helping us through the challenge of infection. It's not a perfect plan; not all bugs, for example, are inhib-ited by heat, and too high a fever will damage you along with the infectious invader. But as a general strategy it seems to work.

These observations suggest that fever-reducing drugs such as aspirin may not always be such a swell idea. It would be ironic if future research concludes that the best thing to do during an illness is simply to endure feeling crummy. But perhaps you'll at least draw some comfort in knowing that, as a result of your stoicism, the pathogen is feeling even crummier.

▶ **ANALYSIS**

1. Create a concept map from the reading, showing how components of the immune system cause the symptoms of a disease.

2. The immune system is a finely tuned, highly responsive system. However, it is also responsible for many of the symptoms of disease. Often, the reason you feel so crummy when you are sick is the result of the immune system doing its job. Write a short essay describing how the symptoms of illness increase your survival advantage. Then describe why or why not you would use symptom-reducing drugs (such as aspirin) when you are sick.

EXTENDING IDEAS

● Research the immune response to a bacterial infection. Compare the immune response evoked by a bacterial infection to that of a viral infection.

● Research the immune response to cancer cells.

● An important feature of the immune system is the ability to distinguish foreign invaders from the body's own cells. Describe the events which occur during immune rejection of organ transplants. Research drugs designed to stop rejection and describe how they work.

◗ Research the biology of an autoimmune disease. Some examples of autoimmune diseases include diabetes, multiple sclerosis, lupus, and arthritis. Describe the events that occur in the immune system to cause the symptoms manifested by one of these diseases, and look for any recent research which is trying to develop ways of alleviating these symptoms.

◗ Some research suggests that the psychological state of an individual may play a role in his/her ability to fight off disease. The implication is that mental functions may be interconnected with the immune system and that the number of lymphocytes may actually increase with a positive outlook. Describe the evidence from sources that suggest this, and evaluate the data.

When a person becomes sick with an infectious disease, a common symptom is swollen glands or lymph nodes. Lymph nodes are part of the lymphatic system of the body. When pathogens enter the body, they eventually make their way into the lymphatic system, where white blood cells live and wage their wars. The lymphatic system also serves as a waste disposal system, filtering out the detritus of the battle. Research the lymphatic system, its components and the ways in which it carries out its functions.

ON THE JOB

PHYSICIAN   Are you a strong problem-solver, who also likes to work with people? Physicians diagnose and treat diseases and disorders of the human body and often specialize in one aspect of medical care. General practitioners see patients of all ages, to diagnose illnesses not severe enough to require a specialist and then prescribe medicine for treatment. Some general practitioners may perform surgery, although most of the time surgery is a specialization. As medicine has become more complex, various specialties have arisen, with physicians continuing their general medical training to concentrate on one area. It can take physicians almost fifteen years to complete their training. This includes a four year college degree (possibly with a pre-medical focus), four years of medical school (the first two years are coursework and the majority of the last two years are spent in a hospital). After receiving a medical degree, physicians complete an internship or residency which can range in length from one year to several years; then many spend an additional 3-5 years learning about one aspect of medical care. One such specialty is that of the allergist-immunologist. These doctors see patients who have a disease or condition caused by allergies, have a problem related to the immune system, or are undergoing surgical transplantation of an organ that may be rejected by their bodies.

General practitioners may work in a private practice, a teaching hospital, or a health maintenance organization (HMO). Physicians may also work in an academic setting (teaching those who are training to become physicians), in a teaching hospital, or in medical research laboratories. Classes such as social studies, math, biology, chemistry, physics, humanities, English, foreign languages and particularly Latin are useful.

BIOLOGICAL TECHNICIAN   Would you be interested in using your organizational and detail-oriented skills to work in a variety of settings? Biological technicians assist biologists in their study of living organisms. The work of a biological technician may be as diverse as biotechnology research and development, pharmaceutical or medical research, or forensics (in police crime laboratories). Biotechnology research and development might result in the development of new products for fields such as medicine or agriculture.

One growing field within biotechnology is monoclonal antibody research. In this research, B cells which secrete a specific antibody are cloned to make multiple copies of the B cell and the antibody. These antibodies can then be used either to stimulate the cell-mediated response into destroying the target cell or used as a "carrier" to take a substance to its target cell. Technicians in this field might clone B cells and their antibodies, attach radioactive molecules or therapeutic drugs to the antibodies which can then be injected into the patient and carried to the target cells, or set up procedures for the manufacturing of monoclonal antibody products. Monoclonal antibody research is also important to pharmaceutical and medical research; it may help lead to cures for AIDS, cancer and other diseases. Depending on the nature of the research, biological technicians might work with laboratory animals such as mice, rats or guinea pigs. With a high school diploma, one year of technical training is necessary for a position as a biological technician. With additional training, technicians can advance to positions as higher level technicians or supervisors. Classes such as biology, chemistry, physiology, math, and English are recommended.

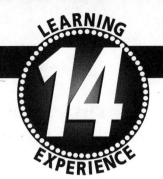
SEARCH FOR THE CURE

Cannon to right of them,
Cannon to left of them,
Cannon in front of them
Volley'd and thunder'd;
Storm'd at with shot and shell,
Boldly they rode and well.
Into the jaws of Death,
Into the mouth of Hell,
Rode the six hundred.

> *Excerpted from* Charge of the Light
> Brigade *by Alfred, Lord Tennyson*

Now that you have explored the infectious microbial world over the course of this module, does this poem reflect your feelings as you step into a room filled with people and all their accompanying infectious companions? Is there anything that we can do to protect ourselves against infectious disease, other than hope our immune system is up to the challenge? In this learning experience, you will be exploring the various ways in which infectious diseases can be prevented and, once contracted, treated. You will then explore the advantages and disadvantages of preventative medicine, such as vaccines, versus taking therapeutic medicine (drugs) in treating infectious diseases in your own life.

An Ounce of Prevention...

With all the reports of infectious diseases appearing in the media, it is perhaps unavoidable, at times, to view the world as teeming with microbes of all shapes, sizes, and ferocities, just waiting for a suitable host—you—to cross their paths so that they can take up residence and literally parasitize the life processes out of you. Reports of outbreaks of age-old diseases, such as cholera and dysentery; the appearance of never-before-identified diseases, such as AIDS and hantavirus; and the recurrence of diseases once thought conquered, such as tuberculosis and staphylococcal and streptococcal bacterial infections—all of these can make you wonder how anyone remains healthy. It's enough to make you avoid eating, drinking, breathing, or touching anything, and certainly enough to make you keep your distance from another person who might be a walking hotel of microscopic menaces.

And yet, many individuals never contract any of these diseases. Many others survive them with few or no physical consequences other than an immunity to reinfection. Clearly, the immune system of individuals plays a role in determining whether, and how sick, an individual may become from an infection. But are there other factors to consider?

Concern about disease and how to deal with it far predates our modern understanding of the causative agents of disease. The search for the cure is as ancient as humankind. Indeed, the healing arts are most likely as old as the martial arts. Almost every society has revered its healers, from the honored medicine men and women in early tribes to the nearly deified physicians in modern society. Early healers usually turned to the natural world for the plant and animal products which seemed to be effective in preventing and treating certain ailments. Even today, modern science still shops at nature's pharmacy. Many of the drugs in common usage have been developed based on the chemical constituents of plants used by traditional healers (see Figure 14.1).

Figure 14.1
Plants are the source of many commonly used medicinal drugs.

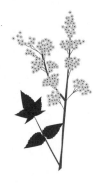 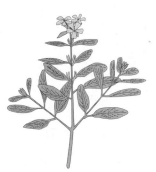 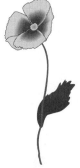 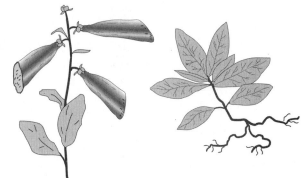

Meadowsweet: Origin of aspirin which reduces pain.

Poppy: Origin of codeine which reduces pain. Also a cough suppressant.

Rosy Periwinkle: Origin of vinblastine which fights cancer.

Foxglove: Origin of digitalis which is used with slow heartbeats or fainting spells.

Ipecacuanha: Origin of ipecac: which induces vomiting.

The old adage "an ounce of prevention is worth a pound of cure" speaks directly to the two major approaches taken in a search for the cure of any disease, prevention and treatment. Prior to the understanding of how infectious disease was spread, prevention was practiced largely on the basis of superstition and tradition. When this approach was effective, it was most likely because traditions and superstitions are often based on generations of observations about what constitutes sensible and healthy behavior. The discoveries that disease could be carried by microbes, and that microbes could be carried through food and water systems, led to a major breakthrough in the prevention of disease. Public health practices have contributed enormously to reducing epidemics of infectious disease. For example, providing clean water and adequate sanitation facilities, regulating procedures for handling food, and educating people about personal hygiene and behavior have greatly lowered the incidence of countless diseases such as plague, cholera, and tuberculosis that decimated populations before the twentieth century.

VACCINES: FOOLING MOTHER NATURE?

In 1796, an English physician, Edward Jenner, made an observation that led to the development of the first vaccine. Smallpox was a terrible disease, widespread throughout history and around the world. Survivors of smallpox were often left with disfiguring pockmarks on their skin, a result of lesions caused by the infecting virus. Because of the prevalence of this disease, scarred individuals were commonplace. Jenner noticed that milkmaids, on the other hand, rarely had pocked skin. He observed that these milkmaids were often in contact with cows infected with a related disease, cowpox, and he hypothesized that this contact protected them from contracting smallpox. Jenner tested his theory by scratching the skin of healthy individuals (starting with his own son) with

Figure 14.2
An 1802 cartoon "The Wonderful Effect of the New Inoculation!" satirizes Edward Jenner and his vaccine against smallpox *(from* Viruses *by Arnold J. Levine, Scientific American Library, New York, 1992).*

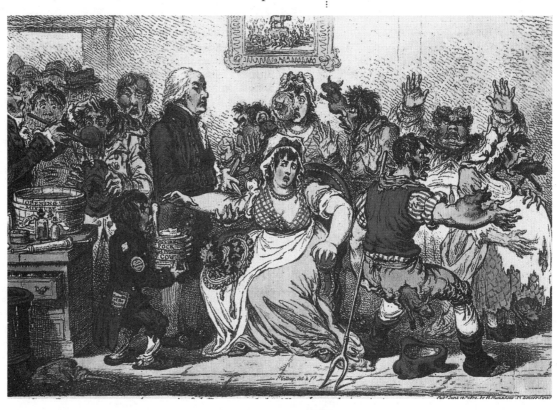

scrapings from cowpox lesions. Crude though they were, these first vaccinations provided effective protection against smallpox. Modern scientific investigations have demonstrated that those scrapings from cowpox lesions contained a virus closely related to the variola virus, the causative agent of smallpox. Though Jenner is credited in the Western Hemisphere with the initial observations about cowpox and with the development of vaccines, the Chinese were carrying out a form of intranasal vaccination for smallpox 1000 years ago; and scarification (scratching the surface of the skin) in India a few centuries later served as Jenner's model for vaccination.

Today, due to an extensive and aggressive vaccination plan around the world, smallpox has been eradicated and has been declared a conquered disease. The only remaining smallpox viruses are samples found in freezers in two laboratories in the United States and in Russia. Much scientific and ethical debate has taken place over whether these stocks of virus should be destroyed. A recent decision (1996) to destroy all remaining stocks will render the smallpox virus truly extinct.

Modern science and technology have developed vaccines for a number of different diseases. Many individuals have been vaccinated against such childhood diseases as measles, mumps, rubella, polio, diphtheria, pertussis, tetanus, hemophilus influenza, and hepatitis. Vaccination is based on the principle that once the immune system has encountered an infectious agent, the system can respond much more rapidly to a repeat exposure to that agent. After the first exposure, it takes about five to seven days for antibodies to appear and nearly two weeks for a full antibody response to develop. A person who has been exposed previously to the agent, however, mounts an antibody response within one or two days because the memory B cells are ready and waiting. Vaccines are designed to confer the benefits of this rapid antibody response without the individual having to endure a full-blown infection and accompanying disease symptoms. A *vaccine* can be made up of one of several different kinds of materials:

- It may be an infectious agent which has been killed and therefore cannot cause a disease.

- It may be an agent whose virulent properties have changed, or mutated, such that the organism can grow but cannot cause symptoms of the disease.

- It may consist of parts of the infectious agent, the antigens to which the immune system responds during an actual infection.

In each of these cases the immune system recognizes the antigens and responds as though the vaccine material were an actual infection.

Although developing a vaccine may sound easy in theory, it can be very difficult in practice. The immune system may recognize that the material in the vaccine is not quite the real thing, and develop a weaker immune response than it would in a real infection. In some cases, components of the vaccine cause the individual to feel sick and suffer side effects. It can be very expensive to develop an effective vaccine ($100–200 million for each vaccine). If vaccines are to make a substantial contribution to public health, they must be available cheaply and readily to millions of people. Despite the obvious long-term gains of preventing disease, at times, economics can block the development and use of vaccines.

▶ ANALYSIS

Write responses to the following questions in your notebook.

1. Describe any experiences that you or anyone you know has had with different kinds of preventative medicine. Can you verify that this behavior or substance prevented the disease? Explain.

2. Using what you know about protein interactions and the immune response, speculate as to why inoculating an individual with the cowpox virus was an effective method in preventing smallpox which is caused by a different but related virus.

3. Describe how a vaccine against cholera might be developed. How would it work?

4. What kinds of vaccines do you think we need to develop today? Explain your decision.

WHEN GOOD THINGS HAPPEN TO BAD BACTERIA

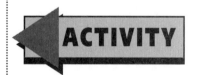

INTRODUCTION   Before the discovery of antibiotics, bacterial infections simply ran their courses. Either the immune system of the patient successfully fought them off and the patient lived to tell the tale, or the patient died. With the discovery of antibiotics, humans felt they had triumphed over microbes. However, the feeling of superiority did not last long.

Within one or two years of the discovery of penicillin, the first drug-resistant strain of staphylococci appeared. As fast as new antibiotics were discovered, resistant strains of microbes were also discovered. Nearly all disease-causing bacteria known to medical science have become resistant to at least one antibiotic, turning a medical miracle into a medical dilemma.

In this activity you will compare the effect of several antibiotics on two non-pathogenic strains of the Gram-negative bacteria *Escherichia coli*. The *Gram stain* technique is a first step in identifying bacteria. The results of this technique will place bacterial cells in one of two groups: Gram-positive bacteria stain deep purple, Gram-negative bacteria stain red. The differential staining reflects differences in the cell walls in these organisms. The cell walls of Gram-negative bacteria have a high lipid content but the cell walls of Gram-positive bacteria have no lipids. The differences in the two groups of bacteria are also reflected in their sensitivity to certain antibiotics, as shown in the table 14.3:

Table 14.3

* Bacteriostatic means the antibiotic prevents bacteria from growing. Bactericidal means the bacteria is killed directly.

ANTIBIOTIC	EFFECT ON BACTERIA*	MODE OF ACTION	EFFECTIVE AGAINST
ampicillin	bactericidal	inhibition of cell wall synthesis	broad spectrum (gram-positive and gram-negative)
tetracyline	bacteriostatic	inhibition of protein synthesis	broad spectrum
erythromycin	bacteriostatic	inhibition of protein synthesis	gram-positive

▶ MATERIALS NEEDED

For each pair of students:
- 2 pairs of safety goggles
- 2 nutrient agar plates
- 1 inoculating loop or sterile cotton swab
- 1 sterile forceps or tweezers
- 1 Bunsen burner or candle
- 1 wax marking pencil
- tape
- distilled water

For the class:
- 2 cultures of *Escherichia coli* bacteria grown overnight (labeled #1 and #2)
- 37°C incubator (optional)
- paper disks soaking in distilled water or one of three antibiotic solutions
- antibacterial solution
- sponges

▶ PROCEDURE

1. **STOP & THINK** Before conducting this experiment, read through the whole procedure. With your partner, design and set up a control for the experiment.

2. Wash your laboratory table with an antibacterial solution. Use sterile procedures as you conduct this investigation.

3. Obtain two nutrient agar plates. Label one #1 and the other #2.

4. Sterilize an inoculating loop in a flame or use a sterile cotton swab. Dip the loop or swab in *E. coli* bacteria culture #1. Remove the cover on a sterile nutrient agar plate. Use the sterile loop or swab to inoculate the agar plate with the bacteria by streaking the bacteria following the same techniques as in Learning Experience 2. Streak the whole plate. Use Figure 14.4 as a guide for the streaking pattern.

5. Repeat the process in step 4 for *E. coli* culture #2.

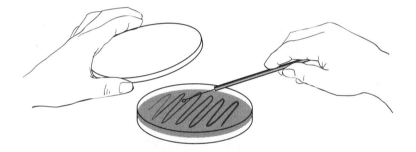

6. Use tweezers to remove two paper disks from each of the antibiotic solutions, and two untreated disks for controls. Place one of each treated disk and one untreated disk in a different part of each of the bacteria-streaked plates. (Be sure to place the disks on areas that you have streaked with bacteria.) Replace covers and secure with tape.

7. Use a wax pencil to mark the location and name of each antibiotic disk on the cover of each plate with the antibiotic being tested. Make a drawing of each plate with appropriate labeling in your notebook.

8. Leave at room temperature to incubate for at least 24–48 hours, or place in a 37°C incubator overnight.

9. After 24–48 hours, when abundant growth on the plates has appeared, examine each plate, and describe and record your observations on each part of the plate. Compare the amounts of growth around the three disks. Measure and record the size of any clear zone, and examine it for any bacterial growth. Record the location and appearance of any growth that you observe inside the clear zone.

Figure 14.4
Procedure and pattern for streaking a plate

▶ ANALYSIS

1. Write a laboratory report for this investigation in your notebook. Be sure to include:
   - the question being asked;
   - the experimental approach you used;
   - the controls you included and why;
   - the results that you observed;
   - any possible sources of error;
   - your conclusions based on your observations;
   - your explanation of what happened at the molecular level.

2. Write a letter to the editor of a health magazine describing how the public must help to combat the impending disaster of antibiotic resistance. This letter should include:
   - a brief overview of the biology of antibiotic resistance;
   - the effects of the development of antibiotic resistance on the emergence of diseases once considered "conquered" and the consequences of this resistance;
   - an analysis of how consumer use and misuse has resulted in deadly consequences;
   - and what steps could be taken to combat this problem by the public and by the medical community.

READING ➤

. . . Is Worth A Pound Of Cure

For a variety of reasons, the prevention of disease may not be possible or may not be the method of choice. In many countries where the majority of people live at a subsistence level, the installation of good sanitary facilities, even to prevent the spread of water borne diseases, seems too costly a burden for their governments to undertake. In some instances, a change of behavior could prevent disease, but changing the personal habits of a lifetime or the cultural habits of generations can be difficult. The process of vaccinating large populations, or for that matter simply getting individuals to sites where the vaccine can be administered, can be very difficult even in cases where effective vaccines exist (and for many diseases, there are no vaccines). In addition, many vaccines require two or more sequential injections. Finding the same individuals again in order to complete the series of injections poses problems, particularly in rural areas. Obtaining sterile needles and providing the storage facilities and refrigeration needed for preventing the denaturation of the protein components of the vaccine can be a logistical nightmare in many developing countries.

Another, less-acknowledged problem with prevention of disease is its lack of drama. Prevention, which results in the absence of disease, is often difficult to appreciate—while the herbal healer or internist who snatches a patient back from the jaws of death is highly praised, appreciated, and rewarded. In many societies the motivation for the development of preventative measures may be less rewarding than discovering the cure.

NEED A HANKY, ALEX?

The "cure" generally takes the form of medicinal drugs. Drugs, in this case, are defined as substances given to humans or animals for the treatment of a disease. A drug may be designed to alleviate the symptoms or it can be used to cure the disease. A drug of the former type can be as simple as the water and salt solution which is the most effective way of treating cholera. This simple solution rehydrates the body and enables the individual to survive the course of the infection by treating the symptoms. Treating the symptoms rather than the cause enables the immune system to establish a response that can clear the infection. For certain viral diseases—colds, influenza, and chickenpox, for instance—bed rest, fluids, and perhaps an occasional bowl of chicken soup, are the best

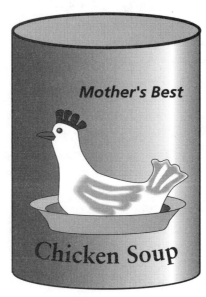

Figure 14.5

and only effective treatments known to date. By taking in nutrients and conserving energy, stricken individuals can assist their immune systems to overcome the unwelcome invader.

Some drugs work directly on the causative agent, in many cases by blocking some specific metabolic function of the organism. The best known example of this type of medicinal drug is the class known as antibiotics. (You encountered antibiotics in Learning Experience 3—Agents of Disease.) Antibiotics are chemical compounds that kill or inhibit the growth of bacteria. They are produced by microorganisms such as bacteria and mold. The story of antibiotics began in 1929, with the British bacteriologist Alexander Fleming. Fleming found that a culture dish in which he was growing *Staphylococcus* bacteria had become contaminated by the fungus *Penicillium*. (Legend has it that Fleming had a bad cold while he was conducting these experiments and the original contaminating organism dripped from his nose.) Rather than just ditching his culture plate in frustration, Fleming took a closer look. He noticed that growth of the staphylococci had been inhibited in the region bordering the mold, as the result of some chemical substance diffusing outward from the mold (see Figure 14.6).

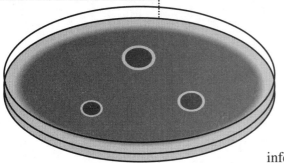

Figure 14.6
Seeing a clear region in the bacterial growth around the mold, Fleming thought the mold was producing a chemical substance that could kill bacteria.

This observation led to the isolation, purificatio and full-scale production of penicillin. When the full potential of such an antibacterial agent was realized, a systematic search for other antibiotics was initiated. Within a few years, a whole medicine chest of different kinds of antibiotics, many isolated from a wide variety of molds and bacteria, was discovered. Medical practice was revolutionized; the bacterial infections which had been among the most dreaded scourges of humankind, such as tuberculosis, syphilis, bacterial pneumonia, and bubonic plague, became treatable. Many scientists and medical practitioners thought that tales of bacterial infections would soon be relegated to the history of science. Little did they realize . . .

ANTIBIOTICS: PROBLEM-SOLVERS OR PROBLEM-CAUSERS?

How do antibiotics work, and how do bacteria become resistant? Penicillin kills bacteria by binding to an enzyme that helps bacteria synthesize cell walls during growth and cell division. The binding of the antibiotic to the enzyme prohibits the bacteria from dividing properly and the bacteria die. Other antibiotics have other targets. Erythromycin binds to a protein of the bacterial ribosome and blocks protein synthesis; tetracycline also interferes with bacterial protein synthesis by binding to the site on the ribosome where tRNAs normally bind; sulfonamides inhibit an enzyme in a synthetic pathway for a compound essential to the synthesis of nucleic acids in bacteria. These compounds bind specifically to bacterial proteins, leaving the host molecules unaffected.

In 1945, Fleming correctly predicted that human behavior leading to misuse and abuse of penicillin would create serious medical problems involving the development of bacterial resistance to the antibiotic. He had already demonstrated in the laboratory that mutants (organisms with altered proteins) present in populations of bacteria were resistant to penicillin. These mutants could be selected for by growing the bacteria in increasingly higher concentrations of the drug. It was later shown that bacteria can develop resistance to penicillin in two ways: (1) A bacterial mutation in an enzyme involved in cell wall synthesis can occur such that the enzyme can still perform its function but no longer binds penicillin. (2) Some bacteria have acquired the capacity to destroy the antibiotic before it destroys them. This can occur when the bacteria acquire new DNA from their environment—DNA that has information for antibiotic-destroying enzymes encoded in it. Where would this DNA come from? Bacteria which make antibiotics would most likely carry genes encoding proteins to protect themselves against the effects of that antibiotic. A current theory hypothesizes that fragments of DNA can contaminate preparations of antibiotics as they are isolated from organisms which produce them. The DNA is carried along as the drug is prepared and ingested, and the DNA fragments are taken up by the bacteria in the body (see Figure 14.7).

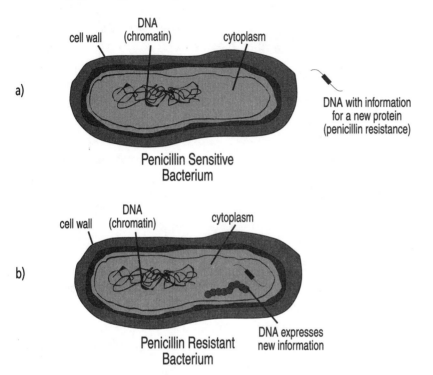

Figure 14.7
Bacteria can take on new characteristics—penicillin resistance, for example—by taking up DNA that contains information for new proteins (such as a protein that destroys penicillin).

What constitutes the misuse of antibiotics? A resurgence of tuberculosis, and the appearance of multi-drug-resistant forms of the bacteria causing it, have been attributed to failure of infected patients to take antibiotics for the entire period of time recommended. When antibiotics are prescribed, an indicated course of treatment is given. Often, upon feeling better, a patient will stop taking the drug, and this can set the scene for a selection of drug-resistant forms of the bacteria.

Drug misuse also arises out of the view that these drugs are a cure for all ills. The patient who has the flu yet insists on a prescription for antibiotics is a common occurrence in doctors' offices around the United States. In many countries antibiotics are available without prescription and are commonly used as self-prescribed cures for all kinds of aches and pains, or as preventative medicine. All of these situations have led to the potentially deadly scenario—that of drug-resistant bacteria causing unstoppable, lethal infections.

With their ability to mutate so readily and with the capacity to shuttle DNA encoding multi-drug resistance back and forth among themselves, will bacteria rule the world in the end? Medical science has marshaled its forces and is taking up some of the same weapons the bacteria use, modification and change.

In the search for new and effective drugs against disease, some scientists have employed a systematic screening of many different kinds of microbes for substances demonstrating antibacterial activity. Others have used a "pull everything off the shelf and try it" approach; this has also proven effective, though tedious and time-consuming. With either method, finding any substance that is even slightly effective gives chemists a place to start, but they may as well be trying to unlock a lock by using every possible key they can find and hoping one works. These approaches have been shown to be expensive and labor-intensive. For each successful drug developed, thousands more have been made and tested. However, in the quest for new antibiotics a combination of these approaches has led to the discovery that certain frogs, moths, pigs, jellyfish, and sharks all contain powerful antibiotics. Researchers are studying these compounds, modifying them and testing them, to determine whether these drugs will serve as a new source of artillery against bacterial diseases.

DESIGNER DRUGS

Another, more rational, approach is being used in the development of "designer drugs." (Recall Learning Experience 8—The Cholera Connection in which you designed a drug against cholera toxin.) It is based on an understanding of the infectious agent, and more specifically of target molecules within that agent, such as enzymes that are required for an essential function. If the structure of the target protein and the process by which it interacts with another molecule are known, then a drug can be designed to compete for the binding site on the target.

This technique is being used in attempts to develop an effective drug against AIDS. An HIV protein, a protease, is required for the virus to process or cut its proteins to the proper size. Drugs are being designed to compete for the binding site of this protease and thereby inactivate it; the proteins required for virus growth would not be available and the virus would be eradicated. Clinical trials currently underway and preliminary data suggest that this drug, in combination with other drugs aimed to fight against HIV, are effective in reducing or eliminating the virus from infected patients. Although early results are encouraging, the long-term efficacy of this approach remains to be determined.

A designer drug approach to developing new antibiotics might involve understanding how an enzyme capable of destroying the antibiotic works and then designing a molecule that fits into the binding site of the enzyme, thus incapacitating its antibiotic-destroying ability.

The causative agents of disease contain many potential target molecules that are unique to that organism, making it possible to develop drugs that kill the agent but leave the host untouched. However, this approach requires in-depth understanding of the biological and biochemical mechanisms of these causative agents and how they cause disease. In addition, the cost of developing these designer drugs is high and is, inevitably, reflected in the final price of the product. This could make the cost of such drugs in developing countries prohibitive.

TAKE TWO FLOWERS AND CALL ME IN THE MORNING

For centuries, the study of plants has led to the discovery of medicines effective against a variety of ills. Curare, used by natives in the Amazon to make deadly poison arrows, is used as a muscle relaxant by surgeons. Young leukemia victims are treated with vincristine and vinblastine, isolated from the rosy periwinkle plant of Madagascar, and taxol, derived from the Pacific yew tree, has been shown to shrink cancer tumors. Quinine, isolated from the cinchona plant, is one of the most effective treatments for malaria. Even the common dandelion, soaked in a little honey, can be eaten to help combat the flu. The croton plant, a colorful plant of Central America commonly used decoratively in American homes, has been used in many parts of South and Central America to make a medicinal tea for cold and flu. (One U.S. drug company has isolated an active compound from the croton plant and is testing it as an oral drug for respiratory viral infections and as a topical ointment for herpes infections.)

The microbial world will forever be a part of the human world. For the most part, the relationship between these worlds is beneficial. However, for adversarial interactions, the battle will be ongoing. Despite immune systems equipped to defend, vaccines designed to protect, and drugs developed to destroy microbes, the microbial world is constantly evolving, changing, and surviving.

▶ ANALYSIS

Write responses to the following questions in your notebook.

1. Describe how bacteria might develop resistance to the drug tetracycline.

2. Describe the steps which might occur when a bacterium takes up a fragment of DNA containing information for drug resistance and explain how this information is expressed.

3. Some scientists argue that humankind will always be plagued by bacteria; drugs offer only a temporary reprieve from suffering, and the only rational approach to defeating infectious disease is with vaccines. Do you agree or disagree with this statement? Explain your answer.

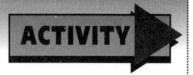

A Shot in the Dark?

INTRODUCTION   To be vaccinated or not to be vaccinated; that is the question faced by many individuals today. Although vaccines have been shown to be very effective against many diseases of childhood, many parents harbor anxieties over whether to have their children vaccinated. In some cases they worry about the side effects, in others the problem is not recognizing the importance of prevention. Because many of these diseases, such as whooping cough, measles, and mumps, are not often seen today because of the availability of vaccines, many parents fail to recognize them as diseases which cause sickness and sometimes death.

In the following article, writer Diane White suffers over making her own decision about whether to be vaccinated against flu. Read her arguments and then carry out the Task.

Flummoxed by the Flu

Diane White, The Boston Globe, December 6, 1993

This year I decided not to get a flu shot. Last year I skipped it. In late winter I came down with something that may have been a kind of flu, but it wasn't bad.

Some people really need flu shots, people in high-risk groups—health care workers, the chronically sick, elderly people. I'd read the news stories reporting a shortage of flu vaccine this year; some people who need shots can't get them. I hated to think I'd be depriving someone who really needed the vaccine.

Then one evening, skimming a magazine and half-watching the news on TV, I heard a voice edged with panic cry, "The worst flu season in two decades!" It was an ad for some patent nostrum alleged to relieve flu symptoms. Night after night I kept seeing the same ad, and the more I saw it, the more difficult it was not to leap to my feet and run to the nearest drugstore to stock up, assuming I could find any. The ad is so persuasive—or manipulative—I wouldn't be surprised if the stuff sold out as soon as the spot aired.

No wonder there's a shortage of vaccine, I thought. No wonder people are clamoring for it. They've all seen that ad.

I decided I'd better get a flu shot.

Watching the ad had made me recall the Hong Kong flu of 1968–69, one of the worst in recent memory. I remembered lying in bed with a high fever, too weak to move, my throat so sore I couldn't talk, every millimeter of my body aching. If the Hong Kong flu did that to me when I was young and healthy, what would it do to me now that I'm middle-aged and broken-down?

Flu shots were being given free at work. The company had a supply, so it wouldn't be as though I were taking it from people who might die if they didn't get it. But how could I be sure? And then I remembered I'd been sick for three days after the last time I'd had the vaccine. Not desperately sick, the way I was with the Hong Kong flu, but sick enough.

I decided maybe I wouldn't get a flu shot.

I'd take a chance. I'd been reading the flu-related stories in the paper. This year's indeed may be the worst in 20 years.

Then again, it may not be. Each year scientists try to predict the exact nature of the influenza virus so a vaccine can be formulated to neutralize it. But the virus mutates so quickly that, by some estimates, they have only a 50–50 chance of being right. So it's a gamble. Flu roulette.

And I'd been reading "A Dancing Matrix: Voyages Along the Viral Frontier" by Robin Marantz Henig, a book both fascinating and humbling. It's fascinating because the subject is compelling and Henig is a superb storyteller, humbling because it puts to rest any notion that human beings control their environment.

Henig writes that many researchers believe we're in for a pandemic of influenza in the next few years. A pandemic occurs when a higher than expected rate of disease strikes several continents at the same time; in an epidemic the higher than normal disease rate is confined to one area. The last pandemic was the Hong Kong flu of 1968–69, which killed 28,000 people, a terrible toll but nothing compared to the 1918–19 pandemic, when between 20 million and 40 million people died.

I decided to get a flu shot. But then I heard Henig in a radio interview. She said that people not in the high risk groups shouldn't get flu shots because the vaccine provides only temporary immunity to a particular strain of flu virus. But if you get the flu, she said, then you'll be immune for life to that strain.

Maybe I wouldn't get a flu shot after all.

Because if I got the flu, I'd be immune for life. Assuming I survived. And what's a week or so of feeling absolutely miserable, with fever and chills and aching all over and coughing and sneezing, compared to a lifetime of immunity to a strain of flu that may or may not come around again?

The next day I got a flu shot.

▶ TASK

Diane White's dilemma over whether or not to get a flu shot is a problem faced by millions of Americans every flu season. In her article she outlines the pros and cons of obtaining a shot. Her arguments acknowledge biological, economic, sociological, and psychological issues. Like Diane White you are to weigh the advantages and disadvantages, or the costs and benefits, of getting a flu shot. One way to approach decision-making is to weigh the possible costs or risks of an action versus possible benefits. Listing the ideas, actions, or outcomes that fall into the two categories can help you decide which plan of action to pursue—or help you identify areas where you don't know enough to make a good decision and need more information. In this type of analysis, remember that a "cost" might not be strictly an amount of money.

An action that wastes your valuable time is a cost. Doing something that would make you sick would be a cost. Similarly, a benefit may be more than having money or a guarantee of good health. A benefit might be something as simple as feeling happy or not having to do something you don't want to do. A benefit might also be a gain for the "greater good" rather than an individual gain.

Set up a table of costs versus benefits on a sheet of paper. Reread Diane White's article, and look for the costs and benefits she weighed in making her decision. Fill in your list with costs and benefits using what you learned about influenza virus in Learning Experience 11 and about the immune system in Learning Experience 13. For example:

▶ COSTS	BENEFITS
Vaccines can make you sick.	Vaccines can keep you from becoming seriously ill.

Make a decision as to whether you would get a flu vaccine and defend your decision. Be prepared to discuss your lists and to address the following in class:

1. I was vaccinated for measles and now I'm immune for life. Why doesn't a flu shot protect me that long? Why do they say I need to have one every year?

2. Isn't the flu that came around two years ago the same as the flu that's making people sick today?

3. Diane White may be able to get one free at work but I have to go to the doctor and it costs a lot of money. Why does it cost so much?

4. I had the flu and my doctor wouldn't give me antibiotics. Why don't antibiotics work against the flu? He told me the only thing to do was to go home, get lots of bed rest, and drink plenty of fluids. My mother could have told me that.

5. I guess I should get a flu shot. Everyone else is getting one.

EXTENDING IDEAS

▶ Your research team at Drugs R Us Pharmaceutical Company has been given the assignment of curing influenza once and for all. You have a budget of several million dollars and the latest in up–to–date technology and equipment. But the team has been deadlocked in a tiny office for weeks arguing over whether the effort should be spent on developing a vaccine or designing a drug. The team is split 50–50 and the arguments are strong on both sides. Describe the costs/benefits of each approach and make the deciding vote on which way the team should go. Explain why you voted as you did.

▶ Mr. C. was a respected businessman from Buenos Aires, who had accumulated a fortune from his family inheritance and personal investments. An energetic man, he spent more than two-thirds of his day pursuing business ventures. He did not like to be held back by sore throats and mild cold symptoms. He generally treated himself with readily available drugs that he bought at the local pharmacy. On one occasion, however, Mr. C. had an exceptionally bad cough and fever, on and off for several weeks. During this time he took several different antibiotics, but nothing seemed to help. Mr. C.'s doctor was concerned and asked him what he had taken. Mr. C. mentioned several, including chloramphenicol, which has been implicated in shutting down blood production in the bone marrow and even causing leukemia. Mr. C. was flown to Boston where he was diagnosed with acute leukemia. He was treated for leukemia using drugs that destroy many of the white blood cells in the body (including T cells and macrophages). Even as the leukemia was being brought under control, his infection raged out of control. The intern told Mr. C. that a common intestinal bacterium, *E. coli*, was circulating in his blood and it was resistant to eight antibiotics. (Normal *E. coli* would be killed readily by any one of the eight.) On the twenty-second day after admission, with his bone marrow free of detectable leukemia, Mr. C. died of bleeding and over-whelming infection. An autopsy revealed that the resistant *E. coli* had produced multiple sites of infection in his liver and other organs. What happened to Mr. C. and why? (*Adapted from* The Antibiotic Paradox *by Stuart B. Levy, Plenum Press, 1992*).

ON THE JOB

LAWYER   How do people protect their inventions and discoveries from being stolen? Lawyers or attorneys are trained to represent either the state or a client in the laws that govern society. It is their job to help clients understand their rights under the law and then to attain these rights in a court of law or government agency. Lawyers may work for businesses, advising on legal matters, helping inventors to secure patents, arranging for stock to be issued, or consulting on tax matters or real estate dealings. They may also work for individuals, advising on buying or selling a home, drawing up wills, or acting as a trustee or guardian. The training lawyers receive and the subsequent licensing allows them to practice law in any area, although many lawyers specialize in one type of law. Not all lawyers work in a courtroom, and not all of a lawyer's time is spent in a courtroom. Many hours of preparation work takes place before a trial. Attorneys specializing in patent law help individuals or corporations to protect an idea or an invention. A background in science may be useful, as some lawyers work for biotechnology companies and need to understand how a company's product or potential product is different from what currently exists. Some lawyers may hold positions as researchers or professors in law school, and some use their training in law in business positions or in governmented agencies. A high school degree, four year college degree, and three years of law school are needed to be a lawyer. Before being allowed to practice in any state, a lawyer must pass the bar (an exam) of that state. Classes in biology, English, and history are useful.

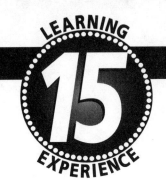

STOPPING THE EPIDEMIC

PROLOGUE **S**ometime in January of 1991, a Chinese freighter arrived in Peru and moored in Lima's harbor. The freighter unloaded its cargo. Then, like so many other vessels in hundreds of other ports around the world, in the quiet of the night it dumped the raw sewage stored in its bilge into the waters of the harbor. Perhaps it was this Chinese vessel—or perhaps another vessel from another part of the world—whose bilge water was teeming with a newly mutated strain of cholera. Perhaps the cholera bacteria were ingested by shellfish in the harbor. Or perhaps those shellfish were harvested by local fishermen, consumed by people in the streets. How the bacteria found their way into the destitute shanty towns of Lima is a matter of speculation. It will never be known for certain. What is known is that by February 23, 1991, Peru's first confirmed case of cholera in almost a century had appeared in a Lima hospital. Soon, physicians would christen the new strain *Vibrio cholerae 01*, serotype Inaba, biotype "El Tor." By the end of 1993, with no end in sight, "El Tor" would cause close to a million cases of cholera, and over 8,600 deaths.

While cholera has made a new home for itself in Latin America, it has always been a part of life in Southern Asia. For generations, it has been *endemic* (constantly present in a location) to regions of India. In more recent decades, it has become endemic throughout Africa as well.

As you have learned in this module, John Snow and Edward Koch "solved" the mysteries of cholera more than a century ago. Snow's research showed conclusively that cholera was a waterborne disease, and identified ways in which its spread could be halted; Koch isolated and identified the agent which caused it. Surely, it seems, in the age of antibiotics and laser surgery, prevention of this disease—the very first to be understood using the techniques of modern epidemiology—should be within our capabilities! So why is cholera a permanent plague in so much of the world? Why, now, is it causing so much misery, from Asia and Africa to Mexico and Argentina? Is it possible to stop it?

Seeking the answers to these questions is, of course, worthwhile because the answers might empower us to improve conditions and to save countless human lives. But they are profoundly worthwhile, also, in that they bring to light the extraordinarily complex relationships between the discoveries of science and the human societies in which those discoveries are used, misused, or lost. The story of cholera in Latin America says a great deal about medicine in the 1990s. At the same time, it says even more about the economic, social, political and organizational context which complicate the way that medicine is practiced.

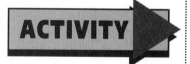

THE TIME OF CHOLERA

INTRODUCTION   In order to dissect the multidimensional problem of cholera, we are going to engage in a role-playing exercise. So imagine, if you will . . .

It is the fall of 1991, and the city of Tumaco, Colombia, is in the early stages of a cholera outbreak. The mayor of the city, in an attempt to bring resources and attention to his people's plight, has initiated a public relations strategy: He has convened Tumaco's first-ever public health conference. Never expecting them to say yes, he has brazenly invited powerful officials from the World Health Organization (WHO), the Pan American Health Organization (PAHO), the Centers for Disease Control and Prevention in Atlanta, GA (CDC), the World Bank, pharmaceutical corporations and politicians from the Colombian National Assembly. To the mayor's surprise, shortly after sending out invitations he receives a phone call from a vice president of the World Bank. The World Bank official wants to know if the conference could be redesigned to focus not just on Tumaco's local problems, but on the spread of cholera throughout Latin America. The mayor responds that the crisis in Tumaco could naturally serve as a model of the problems throughout the continent, and that a focus on Tumaco's local situation would not prevent the conference from also examining the larger issues. He is delighted when the World Bank official answers that in that case, she plans to attend. The mayor is amazed when, after the World Bank official has agreed to attend, one after another, the other powerful invitees phone to say that they, too, will be coming. Though the facilities will be extremely modest, Tumaco now finds itself playing host to a high-powered conference where international data about the epidemic will be examined, and strategies for resolving Latin America's cholera epidemic will be debated and action plans developed.

▶ TASK

Class members are the conference attendees. Collectively, your goals are:

1. to develop an accurate picture of the public health challenges facing Latin America, and then

2. to formulate a plan of action to address those challenges.

The conference itself will take place in two parts such that each of the goals can be addressed fully.

PART ONE

To prepare for Part One of the conference, where the first goal will be addressed, you will have to do all of the following.

1. Carefully read the *Washington Post* article, "The Time of Cholera: One Latin American Town Battles an Epidemic." Also, read the "role profile" notes which your teacher will give you. **Keep your "role profile" secret.** Nobody else should know who you are or what your point of view will be until the conference begins. If a little suspense and mystery are maintained before the conference, it will be more exciting for everyone involved.

2. Develop an opening statement for the conference. The intent of this speech is to share your character's knowledge and concerns with the other conference members. Your speech should last no more than three minutes when you read it aloud. Treat the "character" portion of the profile provided to you as a superficial sketch; your job is to develop that sketch into a complete character, with an identifiable "voice" and perspective. As you develop the voice of your character, consider all of the following questions:

    • What are messages that your character is eager to convey at this conference?

    • Why does your character want to convey these messages? (The messages may be based upon logic, evidence, and idealism and/or the institutional or economic interests of the group she or he represents. Some of the people at this conference have a vested interest in particular outcomes! By the way: having a vested interest does not mean a person is evil.)

    • What kind of information is your character interested in finding out at the conference?

    • What kinds of people is this character likely to choose as political allies? Why?

It is important that you give careful thought to the nature of your character, because for Part Two of the conference, based upon the proceedings in Part One, your character will have to develop an "action plan." The plan will take into consideration what you learned in Part One, but still be consistent with the perspective your character articulated in the first day's discussions. In part, you will be evaluated upon the consistency of your character's voice and perspective. (This does not mean that your character cannot change his or her mind. But if your character came to the conference planning to advocate for children, or seeking government contracts, then he or she should not leave it making a speech about saving the environment and forgetting other issues!)

The Conference

Each part of the conference will be divided into three related portions:
- Medical issues
- Large-scale ("macro") economic and political issues
- Local ("micro") economic and social issues.

Each person will participate in only one portion of the conference but will maintain the same group for Parts One and Two of the conference. For example, if you are preparing to speak as a medical expert during Part One of the conference, you will be responsible only for presenting a medical action plan during Part Two of the conference.

During the proceedings, in addition to making your own speech, you will need to take careful notes while the other presenters are speaking. What they say will influence the action plan that you develop. So if you are speaking about local economic and social problems, you must take notes on what all the other speakers on local economic issues have to say. During the remainder of the conference, you should also be especially attentive, noting any information or ideas, and posing questions that may help you to develop your own action plan.

Part One of the conference will consist of a series of opening statements and question and answer follow-ups. Following each set of statements (for example, when the medical issues speeches have all been made), the entire class will have a chance to ask questions of the speakers.

PART TWO

For Part Two of the conference, the task is to develop an action plan, or policy statement. Once again, this action plan should be presented as a speech. This is a more challenging exercise than preparing the first speech. Now, you must synthesize the sea of information you heard at the conference, and based upon that information, develop an argument for attacking the cholera crisis in a particular way. If you are an expert on large-scale economic and political issues, for instance, your action plan should deal exclusively with these aspects of the crisis.

In your speech, you must answer all of the following questions; in the debate segment of the conference, you must also be prepared to articulate the rationale for each of your policy recommendations.

1. What actions do you think should be taken?

2. Of these measures, which should be done first, second, third, etc.?

3. Prioritize: which measures are most important? Which, least? Could any of these actions be skipped, to save money and or time?

4. Identify the obstacles to carrying out your action plan. If it is to go forward successfully, what pitfalls must be avoided?

5. Identify the likely beneficiaries of your action plan, and those who will probably have to pay for it.

The Conference

Part Two of the Conference will consist of three separate policy debates. Each of the medical experts will present their plans for action; the other medical experts will have an opportunity to challenge or support their peers' proposals. The same process will be repeated for the large-scale (macro) and local (micro) policy groups.

Rules for Conference Proceedings

- Your teacher is the conference moderator. Please respect the moderator's role.

- Raise your hand when you wish to speak. If the moderator calls for order in the conference, please respect this request.

- Fill out a name card with your character's name and title, and place this card in front of your chair at the conference for both sessions. During the conference, be sure to address other conference participants by their formal titles.

► EVALUATION

During one or both parts of the conference your performance may be evaluated by outside guests. Your role-playing will be evaluated on the following criteria:

Part One:

– Is your opening statement clear? Informative?

– Does your opening statement paint a picture of the character and concerns of the individual you are role-playing?

Part Two:

– Is your action plan complete?

– Is it logical and realistic?
  • Does it take into consideration the relevant data which was presented during the first part of the conference?
  • Is there a rationale for the sequence of actions which you will undertake?
  • Have you prioritized your activities?

– Have you identified potential obstacles to success, those likely to pay, and the likeliest beneficiaries?

Overall Evaluation:

You will also receive an overall evaluation for your performance throughout the conference. You will have more information going into Part Two than you had going into Part One of the conference, so you may have changed your mind about many things. However, you will still be evaluated on whether or not your character's underlying perspective has remained consistent over the two sessions of the conference:

– Have the character's priority goals or concerns remained constant?

– Has the character's political perspective remained more or less unchanged?

Your participation in the conference will also be evaluated on:

– When there were opportunities, have you asked questions of other speakers?

– Have you challenged views which contradicted your own or seemed to make no sense?

– Have you respected the other conference members?

– Have you respected the conference process?

The Time of Cholera:
ONE LATIN AMERICAN TOWN BATTLES AN EPIDEMIC

Douglas Farah, Special to The Washington Post, Washington Post Health, *April 23,*

Tumaco, Colombia

One-year-old Sandra Moreno lay motionless in the stifling heat, oblivious to the tube in her arm as her mother gently swept flies away from the baby's gaunt face. In makeshift hospital beds nearby, a dozen listless women, some moaning, lay with intravenous lines protruding from their arms. The cholera ward in the San Andrés Hospital in this rural Pacific coast town is already filled to overflowing; at times, patients are forced to lie on metal stretchers that line the walls. Built as an annex to the hospital auditorium, the 15-bed women's ward is made of cinder block. Its windows are narrow slits without screens; there are neither electric lights nor fans.

Sandra Moreno is among the more recent victims of the cholera epidemic that has killed more than 1,000 people and infected more than 150,000 in Latin America since January. An acutely infectious and potentially fatal disease virtually unknown in developed countries, cholera is spread when food—especially raw fish—and drinking water are contaminated with fecal waste. It is characterized by severe diarrhea, vomiting and fever, which lead to rapid dehydration and wracking cramps.

If too much body fluid is lost, the victim dies, sometimes within hours. Because of the poor sanitary conditions necessary to spread cholera, which is rarely transmitted by person-to-person contact, it is widely known as a disease of poverty.

San Andrés, which treats patients for free, is the only hospital in this high-risk, sparsely populated area of 300,000 people spread over 250,000 square miles. Its resources are already strained to the breaking point although, remarkably, none of the 56 cholera patients who have made it to the hospital so far has died. Local officials attribute its success to the dedication and preparation of the hospital staff.

After a month in which only 40 cases of the disease were reported, in Colombia the number of confirmed cases in the past week jumped to 113, according to health ministry officials; health experts say the epidemic is growing exponentially. "Things are rapidly getting worse, and this is only the beginning, because of the conditions people live in," said Alberto Vargas, director of medicine at San Andrés Hospital. "The water is not fit to drink, the poverty is absolute, and these conditions make Tumaco an area of cultivation of the bacteria. I do not know how we will manage."

Since the epidemic began in Peru last January, Colombia, with more resources and more time to prepare, has been working on teaching its citizens preventive measures, stockpiling rehydration solutions of salts and purified water and making contingency plans to slow the spread and limit the number of deaths, according to Colombia's Health Minister Camilo Gonzalez. Along with educational campaigns that urge people to boil drinking water for 10 minutes, to wash their hands after defecating and to abstain from eating raw fish, the ministry has designed several programs that are just now being implemented.

These include plans to distribute thousands of buckets to be used as toilets, chlorine to purify drinking water and rudimentary treatment of fecal waste.

Although Colombia is better prepared than was Peru, experts agree the epidemic is likely to wreak havoc here and spread through most of the rest of the continent before the year is over. The reason: widespread poverty.

Continued on next page

"Without urgent steps taken in the environment, we will get cholera and more," said Luís Sanchez, an environmental health specialist for the Pan American Health Organization (PAHO). "The technology [of sewage treatment] is available to eradicate these problems, but we do not have the political will or the resources."

THE POOREST REGION IN AN IMPOVERISHED COUNTRY

Tumaco, located on an island, is the center of activity for the Pacific coast region. Its population is predominately black, composed of the descendants of slaves brought over during the nineteenth century to work washing gold scooped from the tropical rivers that criss-cross this area.

This is the poorest region of Colombia. In this city of 60,000 only 8 percent of the houses have any type of sewage treatment, and only about 30 percent have running water. People make their living from fishing, curing hardwoods along the jungle rivers and panning for gold.

San Andrés, a 30-year-old 70-bed hospital is not equipped to handle the new flood of cholera cases, no matter how hard its staff works.

One recent Sunday, a single doctor and two nurses were on duty, tending not only to the nine newly arrived cholera cases but to the many other emergencies that occur in an area already suffering from the peak of the annual malaria season. Health minister Gonzalez said there were 28,000 cases of malaria, a potentially fatal disease borne by mosquitoes, reported along the Pacific coast so far this year.

Even in normal times, the lack of resources makes medical care here difficult. Behind the hospital, where laundry is done by hand, dirty bedding and clothing are piled high. Washing is impossible because the city's faulty water supply often leaves the hospital without water. And when it rains heavily, as it did this month, there is no way to dry clothes, sometimes forcing doctors to delay surgery.

While cholera cases can be fatal and take both time and resources to treat, once a patient starts to be rehydrated, he or she can be cured quickly. Most cholera patients are able to leave after two to three days in the hospital, but that depends on how far dehydration has progressed when they arrive for treatment.

One of the most severe cases to arrive at San Andrés was Pola Quinones, an elderly woman who had suffered from severe diarrhea for three days before her family embarked on the 30-minute canoe ride across the open sea in a driving rain to get her to the hospital. She had been unable to speak for two days, most of her vital signs were extremely weak and her color was a pallid gray.

When she arrived in the hospital, doctors and nurses immediately began rehydrating her through intravenous lines in both arms. As her daughter collapsed in tears in an empty wheelchair, two nurses flanked Quinones and, by hand, squeezed plastic bags filled with fluid to force it into her body more quickly.

After forcing two quarts of fluid into Quinones in less than two hours, they wheeled her to the cholera ward. Two days later, she was able to sit up and drink liquids on her own after receiving almost five gallons of fluid.

"We have to be very aggressive when we get patients like that, or they will die," said Manuel Angulo, a physician at the hospital. "Cholera itself is easy to treat, but the state of shock is what is difficult. If they arrive here with even a little bit of life left, we can save them."

But the Quinones case, along with a dozen others from outlying rural areas, has heightened doctors' fears about the rapid spread of the epidemic.

"We are seeing more and more cases from rural areas, and as that spreads, the difficulty will be in transporting them to where they can be treated," said one medic who asked not to be identified. "That is where we will begin to see our deaths. People can only travel by canoe or on foot and will not make it for treatment."

To help combat the epidemic, the hospital had 30 special beds built. Most are made of wooden planks with a hole cut in the middle and no mattress. That allows patients suffering from acute diarrhea to defecate directly into a plastic bucket, which is then emptied into a special sterilizing solution. To make the beds more comfortable, the hospital experimented with canvas cots with holes cut in them, but the fabric ripped and is costly to replace.

WHY CHOLERA IS FLOURISHING

Three blocks from the hospital, the living conditions that give rise to the epidemic are evident and help explain why cholera is flourishing here.

Houses made of wooden planks sit on platforms far enough above the water to avoid flooding at high tide. At low tide, the beach is piled with trash, which pigs root through while swarms of flies feast on excrement.

In the Las Americas neighborhood, Alfonso Palacios, 60, said he and his family have begun boiling their drinking water, although many of his neighbors have not.

To help explain the difficulties the neighborhood faces, he led visitors on a precarious wooden walkway built on 10-foot stilts over the garbage and water, past crowded houses, to a cement structure missing most of its roof and part of its walls, perched over the ocean.

Palacios explained that the building, which contains eight stalls, is the neighborhood bathroom used by dozens of people. Feces and urine fall straight into the ocean below and are then washed ashore. A few yards away, children splash in the ocean.

"The children love to play in the water," Palacios said. "Often, they get sores on their arms and legs from the swimming, but we cannot stop them."

While many people here say they are boiling their drinking water—in accordance with an announcement broadcast repeatedly on radio and television—others, having received little help from authorities for decades, are suspicious of the measure or simply refuse.

Because diarrhea from parasites and malnutrition is so widespread, Vargas, the medical director of San Andrés Hospital, said that many people here cannot distinguish cholera as a more severe disease than the usual ones with which they are afflicted. Other health experts say that many more victims than the number officially reported may have died without being diagnosed or treated.

"It is difficult for people to accept change here," he noted. "You cannot change centuries of culture in two or three days. It will take years."

In the Vientos Libres neighborhood, two elderly women who sat in the doorway of their raised house chewing sugar cane stalks illustrated Vargas's statements.

"I do not boil my water, and I never will because boiled water tastes different," said the owner of the home, who declined to give her name. "If God wants me to get cholera, I will get it, and if He wants to cure me, then I will not die."

In Las Flores, as with most of the poor neighborhoods, drinking water comes through half-inch water pipes at ground level settled in the permanent mud; when not in use, the pipes are covered with a screw-on plastic cap. Water can only be gathered in buckets during low tide. The houses are built on seven-foot stilts, and when the tide comes in carrying garbage and fecal waste, it covers and fouls the water pipes.

Nearby, three children standing in the mud fill tin pans with ocean water, which they drink, as adults lounge on catwalks above.

"This is the way we live," said Andres Lopez, a local resident. "We have no resources to change."

Continued on next page

"ONLY CATASTROPHE GETS THE GOVERNMENT'S ATTENTION"

While the health of Pacific coast residents has long been precarious, the cholera epidemic has now plunged the economy into decline and has also become a political issue.

Because one of the main ways cholera bacteria is spread is by eating raw fish, Colombia's internal seafood market has collapsed. Scientists say that cooking seafood carefully completely kills the bacteria, but the fear of eating any fish or seafood persists.

Because no evidence of contamination has been found in deep-sea fish or carefully controlled shrimp farms, exports have not suffered.

Dario Garces, owner of Inpespa, one of the largest fish processing plants in Tumaco and president of the city's chamber of commerce, said he had shut down his plant and was precariously close to bankruptcy. He said a recent study by the chamber of commerce showed that Tumaco was losing $167,000 a day in fish sales and the subsequent ripple effect through the small economy.

Ernesto Kaiser, Tumaco's mayor, who is widely respected for his efforts to bring aid to the city, said that he would push the government to commit the millions of dollars necessary to end the threat of cholera by building sewage and water treatment systems. But, Kaiser acknowledged, his chance of success was a long shot.

"Only catastrophe gets the government's attention," Kaiser said. "We need to seize the moment and get the resources now, before we are forgotten again."

Even if Tumaco officials manage to draw attention to their plight, the rest of the coast is far less fortunate, as the experience of the village of Salahonda, an hour ride by launch across the bay, demonstrates.

Roberto Castillo is the only doctor in the swampy town of 6,000 who treats cholera cases that arise among residents who live upriver. "Our case load is doubling every week," said Castillo, who recently treated 25 cases in his 12-bed clinic. "I am exhausted, I have no time to sleep."

Because of the lack of resources, each patient has to bring bedding and food, although treatment is free. There is electricity only from 7 p.m. to 11 p.m., when the generator is working. Just two houses have septic tanks, and raw sewage runs through a ditch in the middle of town.

"My biggest fear is that we will see cholera stay as an endemic disease, as malaria is," Castillo said. "Right now, it costs us about $120 to treat each patient, and the government, because of the emergency, has given us the resources. But that will not last indefinitely, and then what will we do?"

In the nearby hamlet of La Playa, fishermen cut up the day's catch to salt and dry, then sell upriver. Because the fish companies stopped buying fresh fish since the epidemic began, the fishermen work twice as hard for less money.

One old man, sitting on a wooden bench under a shade tree with three friends, said he does not understand why everyone is talking about cholera. "They say that cholera can kill us, and that we can get it from the fish," he said, while his friends nodded in agreement. "But if that were true, then, if the fish had cholera they would die, wouldn't they? That is why I do not believe them."

Asked if he is boiling his water, he laughed. "Boiled water does not quench your thirst," he said. "It is the same as drinking nothing."

Castillo said such responses are normal. Many people here blame cholera not on bacteria but on the "evil eye" or another curse inflicted by an enemy.

"That is why cholera will advance as far as hygienic conditions permit it to go," he said. "And here, that is very, very far."

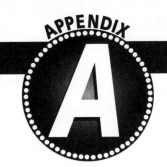

GLOSSARY OF TERMS

The following terms can be found on the listed page in the Student Manual, unless otherwise noted. ◆ indicates pages which you may receive from your teacher.